THE
EVERYTHING®
GUIDE TO
THE BLOOD SUGAR DIET

Dear Reader,

If you're looking to balance your insulin levels, eat healthier, or lose weight, then the blood sugar diet is a great way to get started. Scientists are discovering that the secret to losing weight, maintaining good health, and preventing illness lies in balanced blood sugar—and keeping blood sugar levels in a healthy range isn't just a concern for those diagnosed with diabetes or prediabetes. The blood sugar diet is also effective in preventing obesity, high blood pressure, heart disease, and more.

If you have been diagnosed with diabetes, you know how life altering it can be. Your doctor may give you the option of making a lifestyle change by improving your health with diet and exercise, or prescribing a medication. However, I hope you are reading this book before diabetes has even become an issue, when you realize changing your habits with the blood sugar diet will help you achieve long-term weight loss and in turn reduce your risk of diabetes, as well as the other health issues that come along with it.

My passion and commitment to diabetes and disease prevention is one that hits close to home. My amazing, large, Midwest-rooted family has a history of diabetes, as well as heart disease, cancer, and arthritis. As a registered dietitian focused on metabolism and disease prevention, my goal is to help you and your family, friends, and others on their quest of living a happy, healthier life, free of disease. The goal of the book is to empower you to improve your lifestyle in order to ensure good health in the future. Diabetes and other weight-related health issues do not happen overnight, so do your best to identify your risk early and take the steps to transform your life, reversing their potential onset. This guide will give you the tools and recipes to help you along the way to better health.

Emily Barr, MS, RD

Welcome to the EVERYTHING® Series!

These handy, accessible books give you all you need to tackle a difficult project, gain a new hobby, comprehend a fascinating topic, prepare for an exam, or even brush up on something you learned back in school but have since forgotten.

You can choose to read an Everything® book from cover to cover or just pick out the information you want from our four useful boxes: e-questions, e-facts, e-alerts, and e-ssentials.

We give you everything you need to know on the subject, but throw in a lot of fun stuff along the way, too.

We now have more than 400 Everything® books in print, spanning such wide-ranging categories as weddings, pregnancy, cooking, music instruction, foreign language, crafts, pets, New Age, and so much more. When you're done reading them all, you can finally say you know Everything®!

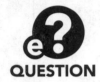

QUESTION

Answers to common questions

FACT

Important snippets of information

ALERT

Urgent warnings

ESSENTIAL

Quick handy tips

PUBLISHER Karen Cooper

MANAGING EDITOR, EVERYTHING® SERIES Lisa Laing

COPY CHIEF Casey Ebert

ACQUISITIONS EDITOR Hillary Thompson

ASSOCIATE DEVELOPMENT EDITOR Eileen Mullan

EVERYTHING® SERIES COVER DESIGNER Erin Alexander

Visit the entire Everything® series at *www.everything.com*

THE
EVERYTHING®
GUIDE TO THE
BLOOD SUGAR DIET

Balance your blood sugar levels to reduce inflammation,
lose weight, and prevent disease

Emily Barr, MS, RD

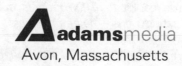

▲adamsmedia
Avon, Massachusetts

*This book is dedicated to all of those who have struggled
with their weight. May this book lead you to the promised
land of better health and extra years of happiness.*

Published by
Adams Media, a division of F+W Media, Inc.
57 Littlefield Street, Avon, MA 02322. U.S.A.
www.adamsmedia.com

Contains material adapted from *The Everything® Diabetes Cookbook, 2nd Edition* by Gretchen Scalpi,
copyright © 2010, 2002 by F+W Media, Inc., ISBN 10: 1-4405-0154-8, ISBN 13: 978-1-4405-0154-8; *The
Everything® Vegan Cookbook* by Jolinda Hackett with Lorena Novak Bull, copyright © 2010 by F+W
Media, Inc., ISBN 10: 1-4405-0216-1, ISBN 13: 978-1-4405-0216-3; and *The Everything® Green Smoothies
Book* by Britt Brandon with Lorena Novak Bull, copyright © 2011 by F+W Media, Inc., ISBN 10: 1-4405-
2564-1, ISBN 13: 978-1-4405-2564-3.

ISBN 10: 1-4405-9255-1
ISBN 13: 978-1-4405-9255-3
eISBN 10: 1-4405-9256-X
eISBN 13: 978-1-4405-9256-0

Printed in the United States of America.

10 9 8 7 6 5 4 3 2 1

Contents

09 Soup Lovers / 141

10 Variety of Veggies / 155

Acknowledgments

I would like to dedicate this book to my family: my soulmate, Clabe, and our two amazing children. You have pushed me into a new reality and have always encouraged me to think outside of the norm. Thank you for giving me the strength to take on challenges that no one in their right mind would, especially a mother of two-year-old twins! Thank you to my parents, my sister, who has moved her way into being my best friend, my brother, sister-in-law, amazing nieces and nephews, and my extended Barr and Gaines family, who have been supportive of all of my accomplishments, dreams, and decisions I have made along the way. This book would never have been possible without all of their support, as well as the support from my Kansas City and Orange County dietitian friends. They have expanded my food repertoire, knowledge, and comfort level with new and intimidating foods, especially on girls' night.

Thank you to Marlayna and The Skinny Gene Project for their devotion to diabetes prevention and believing in me as I help lead their nutrition fight. Thank you to everyone who has taken the time to teach me, especially the physicians and dietitians who taught me the ins and outs of nutrition and metabolism. And a special thank you to Adams Media for giving me this incredible opportunity, guidance, and support.

Introduction

WHILE DIABETES MIGHT BE the first thing you think of when you hear the words *blood sugar diet*, really, this diet is focused on limiting your intake of processed foods to impact your health in a variety of wonderful ways. Diabetes prevention is one obvious goal of the blood sugar diet, but your health benefits certainly won't stop there. The foundations of the blood sugar diet overlap with the prevention of heart disease, cancer, arthritis, inflammation, and ultimately will help you lose weight, which benefits you inside and out. The CDC has said that one in three American adults has prediabetes. This is an alarming realization, especially considering the fact that 90 percent of these people do not even know they have it.

One of the most common red flags for becoming diabetic is family history. Traditionally, diabetes has been something you just accept. You may think, "It runs in my family, so no reason to get worked up over it. It's just the way it is." But as more and more knowledge is gained through research and medicine, this way of thinking is changing.

First and foremost, it is essential to know the risk factors regarding diabetes. If you find that you are predisposed to this condition, you should be evaluated often to see if you are at risk for developing prediabetes. Prediabetes and diabetes are preventable and reversible with the right lifestyle changes.

Of course, the key word is lifestyle. Very often, trying the newest diet program, with its promise of weight loss in a matter of "minutes," seems easier than changing your exercise and nutritional routine. Whether the diet is low-fat, no carbs, high-fat, high-protein, detox, juicing, or whichever combination, you know how it works. The diet includes a very specific set of rules that set up boundaries to help you stay on track. Following a very restrictive diet can result in short-term success but not long-term success. At some point you will decide that you are sick of the diet, or on a positive note, that you are happy with the weight-loss success you have achieved; you start feeling better about yourself, then begin to loosen up your diet restrictions, and soon you bail on the diet and all of its rules to return to your usual life (which may have started the problem in the first place).

The blood sugar diet focuses on a lifestyle free of most processed foods, replacing these boxed items with fresh, whole, natural foods. The foods you consume affect your blood sugar patterns, increasing or decreasing your diabetes risk. By increasing your intake of fiber with foods such as beans, nuts, vegetables, and fruits, your weight will get into balance and your blood sugars will follow suit.

It is especially important to know how to balance out your meals. Each meal should include a high-fiber option to slow down the sugar transfer into the bloodstream, paired with a healthy-fat option to also help slow things down. Protein is vital for the body, but surprisingly, your need is much lower than you may expect. Protein is prevalent in vegetarian sources including beans, lentils, and nuts, and then if you layer in your goal of two servings of fish per week, you should be in pretty good shape. The blood sugar diet will give you the tools to set yourself up for success. You will learn to eliminate the processed items while stocking up on seasonal produce and staples to make meal planning a cinch.

The goal is a lifestyle change. This will not only allow you to avoid the emotional roller coaster ride of your fluctuating weight, but it will also allow you to feel better about yourself. You will be free of the guilt of "eating badly" or "cheating" on your diet. You can't cheat on your lifestyle change if it is set up to support your specific life demands. You will improve your general health while decreasing your risk of diabetes, both beneficial to help you achieve your personal goals. The blood sugar diet will give you the balance to manage your diet while enjoying your life.

CHAPTER 1

Introduction to the Blood Sugar Diet

When you hear the words *blood sugar*, you may automatically think of diabetes. The reality is that type 2 diabetes is the late phase of blood sugar imbalance—the stage when it is out of control. There is a slow transition that occurs as the body moves toward diabetes. The first part of the transition is the healthy phase, when your blood sugars are normal and balanced. Next comes the warning zone (prediabetes), when your blood sugar is high but not high enough to be classified as type 2 diabetes. Eventually, if left untreated, high blood sugars can lead to full-blown diabetes. It is important to know if you are at risk for diabetes, and how the blood sugar diet can help you make over your lifestyle to prevent it. Also keep in mind that this insulin-balancing blood sugar diet is great for *everyone*—and can help you lose weight while preventing and reducing risks of other diseases.

What Is the Blood Sugar Diet?

Here are a few facts about the blood sugar diet:

- This diet is not just for people with diabetes. It is good for everyone, with or without diabetes, and especially for those at risk for diabetes.
- This is not a low-carb diet; this will become clear in the next chapter. You will be eating plenty of carbs, maybe just limiting some of the obvious, not-so-blood-sugar-friendly carb sources.
- This is not a low-fat diet. Fat is your friend, as long as the fat comes from the right sources—mainly plant based and in the right amounts.
- This is not a calorie-counting diet. Choosing the right fiber-filling foods will lead to the goal of lowering your calorie intake and boosting weight loss.
- This is not a vegetarian diet. Although this diet may seem to lean closer to this lifestyle, fish, lean meat, poultry, and small portions of dairy can be incorporated into this eating pattern and the recipes in this book.
- This isn't actually a diet; it's a lifestyle. Shoot for the 80/20 rule, staying on track at least 80 percent of the time and leaving room for splurges.
- This is a heart-healthy diet. It should increase your good cholesterol and decrease your bad cholesterol while keeping your blood pressure in check.
- This is a fiber-rich diet, being that fiber is the foundation for regulating blood sugar, cholesterol, and your weight.
- This is a nutritionally balanced diet. Focus on eating plant-based foods and oils while eating animal-based foods in moderation.
- This is not a restrictive diet. All types of foods can fit into this diet, including gluten and dairy, just in limited amounts.

Your Calculated Risk

On the outside it seems that everybody is different, but in reality, there are three reasons why everyone is at risk for prediabetes or type 2 diabetes. These three components are ethnicity, family, and the environment in which you live; and unfortunately, all three are out of your control.

No matter your ethnicity, you are at risk for prediabetes and type 2 diabetes. You are born with roots and a family tree, and you had no say in the health of your family members. If someone in your family has diabetes, you are automatically at a higher risk of having diabetes yourself.

It is estimated that 86 million people fall into this early diabetic category labeled "prediabetes." This is a nice way of saying you are on your way to diabetes, the seventh leading cause of death in the United States (CDC) and eighth leading cause of death in the world (WHO). But even worse, diabetes is now being linked to increased risk of heart disease and certain cancers, and is said to shorten your life by six to ten years, comparable to the years shaved off life expectancy by long-term cigarette smoking. This information is not intended to scare you, but it is meant to shed light on medical facts that are often swept under the rug. Identifying the early signs of prediabetes and diabetes is actually good, because you can do something about it.

In American society, you are exposed to foods with sugar, fats, and excessive calories on a daily basis. Nearly 70 percent of adults in the United States are overweight or obese. Obesity often goes hand in hand with type 2 diabetes. In fact, 80–90 percent of those with type 2 diabetes are overweight or obese (for more information, visit *www.obesity.org*). There is also an alarming increase in the incidence of prediabetes and type 2 diabetes in American children, which was unheard of in the past as type 2 diabetes was previously referred to as the adult onset disease.

It may seem that the diagnosis of prediabetes and type 2 diabetes is unavoidable, but the reality is that, unlike some other diseases, prediabetes and type 2 diabetes are avoidable and reversible with the proper diet and lifestyle.

For reference, here is a list of diabetes risk factors:

❑ Overweight or obese—calculated body mass index (BMI) > 25
❑ Sedentary lifestyle
❑ Impaired glucose tolerance
❑ Insulin resistance
❑ High blood pressure
❑ Low HDL (good) cholesterol
❑ Over forty-five years old
❑ History of gestational diabetes or polycystic ovary syndrome (PCOS)

How do you calculate your body mass index (BMI)?
Your BMI is a marker to tell you if you are at a healthy weight. To calculate your BMI, first multiply your height (in inches) × your height (in inches). Now divide your weight (in pounds) by your squared height. Take your answer and multiply by 703. An ideal BMI range for healthy adults is 18.5–25. If your BMI number is between 25 and 30, you are classified as overweight. If your BMI is 30 or more, that indicates obesity. Keep in mind that the BMI calculation does not take muscle mass into account. If you were to check the BMIs of many professional athletes, on paper they may appear obese, but in actuality this couldn't be further from the truth!

How Does the Diet Work?

The blood sugar diet is not specifically a diabetic diet; it's actually a weight loss and weight management diet intended to prevent the onset of diabetes as well as other diseases, such as heart disease and cancer, and reduce the inflammatory response of the body (arthritis). If your weight falls into the risky danger zone of overweight or obesity, then this blood sugar–regulating and disease-reduction diet is for you. But this type of eating style is also perfect for most people. Of course, there are some people who have other health issues, and because of this, the blood sugar diet may not be the right diet for them.

When your body is healthy, it is able to process foods and their nutrients efficiently. You eat foods, they are digested as they move through the stomach and intestines, and then the nutrients are absorbed. These nutrients move to the bloodstream in order to be distributed to the right places. Insulin (a hormone) is the key ingredient that moves sugar from the blood to other tissues in your body for energy or to be stored for backup energy. The problem with prediabetes and type 2 diabetes is that the body is unable to move sugar out of the bloodstream. This happens over time: As the pancreas is not able to keep up with the demands of the body (usually from the stress of overeating), the pancreas will not produce enough insulin or the body is not able to use the insulin efficiently to keep blood sugars in a healthy range.

The blood sugar diet is targeted to help your body regulate your blood sugar efficiently to prevent this from happening in your future.

The blood sugar diet focuses on giving your body the right balance and types of carbohydrates, proteins, fats, and water. When your intake of these core nutrients is out of balance, oftentimes it leads to the slowing of your metabolic rate and the increasing of your body's stores of fat.

FACT

Some research out of Virginia Tech has proposed that being only 1 percent dehydrated significantly slows down your metabolic rate. Water is a required agent for a large majority of the metabolic reactions in your body. Therefore, when you are dehydrated, it makes sense that your metabolism may not be functioning at its highest. So drink up!

Reap the Health Benefits

Instead of looking for the sounds-too-good-to-be-true diet, set your goal for healthy, controlled weight loss that is sustainable. The primary goal of the blood sugar diet is to help your body function well, reducing your risk of diabetes. The secondary outcome is that following this type of eating pattern in tandem with regular physical activity will actually cause you to lose weight to achieve and maintain a healthier body weight. This, in turn, will help you achieve the primary goal as well.

Focusing on the core nutrients in the proper balance will maximize your metabolism, which is an amazing benefit for anyone over the age of thirty or those who have seen their metabolism begin to slow. The great thing about eating to control your blood sugar is you are eating in a way that will help you maintain or lose weight. A healthy weight drives a healthy body and metabolism.

There are a few additional health benefits of this diet. First, it is high in fiber, which will help lower your cholesterol. Many foods rich in fiber also happen to be rich in vitamins, minerals, antioxidants, and phytochemicals (all great things!), further reducing your overall risk of cancer.

ALERT

You may feel like you have a free pass with fats and proteins since they do not directly impact your blood sugar in the way carbs do. But the fact of the matter is that extra intake of anything (even if it's healthy!) can and will result in fat storage. The only way to offset this is to burn extra calories to keep your weight in balance. When you are at an unhealthy weight, your metabolism is unhealthy as well.

Making this change to your lifestyle will also reduce your risk of heart disease, which is the number-one cause of death in the United States. Unfortunately, there is a strong relationship between your heart health, diabetes, and obesity. It is important to identify, treat, and, if possible, prevent these life-threatening conditions from becoming part of who you are.

Breakdown of Blood Sugar: It's Quite Simple!

Blood sugar is exactly what it sounds like: the amount of sugar (a.k.a. glucose) floating around in your blood. So what's the big deal about your blood sugar? Blood sugar is an important marker that helps you know how well your body is working. If elevated, your blood sugar can be an indicator that your body may be progressing toward disease (diabetes). You need some sugar in your blood, but it needs to be in a balance. When there is too much sugar in the blood, the body becomes stressed and has to work harder to move the sugar out of your blood to other places in your body where it can be used for energy or stored for later use.

The foods you eat directly impact your blood sugar. The goal is to avoid rapid increases and decreases in blood sugar. The number-one culprit in this process is sugar. This simple carbohydrate is small in structure and is rapidly digested and absorbed into the bloodstream. This causes the pancreas to release insulin rapidly to help move the sugar out of the bloodstream. The blood sugar goes up but just as quickly goes down, which is why you may feel hungry not too long after consuming sugar. This cause-and-effect relationship of the blood sugar rebounding is not so good for your waistline or your heart, as it results in an increase in blood pressure, cholesterol, and triglycerides.

Your blood sugar rapidly going up and then crashing down is exactly what the blood sugar diet prevents. If this situation happens day in and day out, month after month and year after year, you will eventually wear out your pancreas and the sugar will be trapped in your blood. As you can imagine, at this point, your blood becomes a little thicker—think of the high sugar content and consistency of syrup—and has a difficult time moving through your body, especially through some of the really narrow capillary beds. This is why diabetics may have trouble with their eyes, feet, and overall circulation. It also makes the heart work harder to pump the thick, sticky blood throughout the body.

Get Stable, Starting with Avoiding Added Sugar

Foods with added sugar provide non-nutritive calories that pose a huge risk to your health. Not only do they affect your blood sugar control, but they also contribute to weight gain and diseases associated with obesity.

The solution is to pay attention to the foods you are eating. Added sugar is found in many processed foods and sweetened drinks, primarily in the form of sugar and high fructose corn syrup. While these two are the most popular forms, it is important to read nutrition labels and look for the other key words that also mean sugar, usually ending in -ose. Other natural sweeteners such as honey and agave nectar are similar to sugar, as they are rapidly absorbed in the body and can negatively affect blood sugars.

You may have to turn into a detective to catch all of the manufacturers' attempts to hide the added sugar under an alias. Sugar may be added to foods where you least expect it because it has so many functions. Sugar is able to boost up the flavor, improve texture, and preserve foods, which is why processed foods so often contain sugar. You should be sure to check any food that has a label to see if it contains sugar; you may be surprised to find it in ketchup, salad dressings, and even mustard. No processed food is safe.

A good rule of thumb is to avoid foods that include added sugar as one of the first three ingredients. Don't stop reading after the first three ingredients, though. If the food contains several different sources of added sugar positioned anywhere on the ingredient list, you best avoid these foods, too. You may also look at the nutrition facts label to see how much sugar the food contains. This method is a bit tricky, as you need to decide if the sugar is a naturally occurring sugar, as in fruit or dairy foods, or actually an added sugar.

ALERT

The food industry is getting creative, breaking up the amount of sugar added into several ingredients so they are listed toward the end of the ingredient list. This makes them less harmful for us, right? Nice try. Avoid these fraudulent foods with multiple sugars!

Here is a list of common sugar aliases: brown sugar, cane sugar, confectioners' sugar, corn sweetener, corn syrup, corn syrup solids, dextrin, dextrose, evaporated cane juice, fructose, fruit juice concentrates, glucose, high fructose corn syrup, honey, invert sugar, lactose, malt syrup, maltose, maple syrup, molasses, raw sugar, sucrose, sugar, sugar syrup.

It is recommended that you keep your intake of added sugar as low as possible. The American Heart Association recommends limiting your intake of added sugar as follows:

- Men: 150 calories per day = 9 teaspoons or 38 grams sugar
- Women: 100 calories per day = 6 teaspoons or 25 grams sugar

The recommendations for children are based on their calorie requirements. Here are some general guidelines:

- Preschool: 50–70 calories per day = 3–4 teaspoons or 13–17 grams sugar
- School-age (4–8 years): 50 calories per day = 3 teaspoons or 12 grams sugar
- Preteens and teenagers: 85–135 calories per day = 5–8 teaspoons or 21–34 grams sugar

For more infomraiton, visit *http://ndb.nal.usda.gov/ndb/foods.*

A recent report from the American Heart Association found that Americans consume way too much sugar, an average of 20 teaspoons of added sugar per day. This translates into eating 200–300 percent of the recommended amounts of added sugar per day, increasing your calorie intake by 325 calories daily. The NIH has analyzed sufficient evidence to support the conclusion that increased consumption of sugary beverages, including chocolate milk, will dramatically increase your risk of diabetes, and by replacing one sugary beverage per day with water, you will reduce your risk of diabetes by up to 25 percent. Interestingly enough, the artificially sweetened (diet) beverages pose the same risk. The research goes on and on about how to reduce your risk of diabetes. Let's kick the added sugar, artificial sweeteners, the extra weight, and let's not forget to kick processed foods to the curb.

Simple or Complex: Are All Carbohydrates Bad?

The quick answer is no! If you turn that question around, would you consider beans, vegetables, and fruits bad? Obviously not, but let's just face it, with the ever-changing media message, carbs are confusing. Good one day, not good the next, then suddenly carbs are okay again! It really shouldn't be that confusing. Some may think carbs make you gain weight, and they can. You will gain weight if you eat the wrong kinds of carbs and in the wrong amounts. But they can help you lose weight, too, that is if you choose the right types of carbs, in the right amounts.

Focus on the right carbs. Complex carbs are the "good" ones, especially if they are full of fiber. The reason they are complex is that they take longer to break down in the course of digestion; therefore, the body has time to respond to the food without throwing your blood sugar or metabolism out of balance. When you eat these types of carbs, your body will actually send a message to the brain to turn off your hunger; therefore, you will stop eating at the right time. Of course, sometimes you may not listen to that message, but that's another story.

So what should you do about the sugar in dairy and fruits? The sugar in these foods is classified as natural sugar, meaning there is no way around it; the sugar is in there. The important thing to remember about these two food groups is that they also have other nutritional qualities that help keep your blood sugar from spiking. In general, it is safe to say that fruits and low-fat dairy or dairy substitutes are recommended for most people.

Nearly all fruits contain fructose but also provide a good source of fiber, which helps slow down the process of sugar breakdown. If an apple had a nutrition label, you may be surprised to see that this superfood—that keeps the doctor away—actually has 19 grams of sugar but also 4.5 grams of fiber. This amount of sugar is comparable to an 8-ounce glass of Sprite. How is Sprite even comparable to an apple? It's not.

These two foods are quite different; it's all about the source of the sugar and the way the body processes it. The sugar in fruit is natural, compared to the second ingredient listed on the can of Sprite: high fructose corn syrup. Ironically, both of these sugars are considered simple sugars, but they act differently in the body due to the way they are packaged. The sugar in the Sprite is rapidly absorbed into your bloodstream. It's not good for your body to have to respond to a sugar load like this.

Imagine if you had a medium Sprite from a fast-food restaurant. The sugar in this drink would hit your bloodstream with 44 grams of added sugar, which may cause a "sugar high," followed by an awful "sugar crash" (i.e., fatigue). Constantly bombarding your body with rapidly absorbed sugar puts you at risk for some major health problems (diabetes, obesity, high triglycerides, and decreased HDL cholesterol, putting you at risk for heart attack and stroke).

Unlike the added sugar in Sprite, an apple is digested slower due to its fiber content. Therefore, the body is able to handle the sugar while keeping your blood sugars more stable, which is an excellent way to control and/or prevent diabetes.

ALERT

Of course, there is always one exception to the rule: juice. Even if juice or fruit smoothies are labeled "100 percent fruit juice," they still most likely will not contain enough fiber to keep blood sugars from rising rapidly; therefore, the actual fruit is always a much better choice.

Lactose is the sugar found in dairy products. Most people have decreased enzyme activity that makes digesting lactose difficult. Dairy can be a good source of protein and may also contain some fat that will help slow things down as well. Due to the increased manipulation of cow's milk and the fact that it is meant for cows and not humans, it is probably a better option to try incorporating a dairy substitute and a variety of greens and fish into your diet to meet your calcium and vitamin D needs.

Believe it or not, the complex carbohydrates found in foods such as pastas, breads, and cereals all break down into simple sugars as well. The process is much like that of the apple: slow digestion and absorption, resulting in mild to moderate changes in blood sugars. It's especially beneficial to your blood sugar to choose high-quality, whole-grain options that include more fiber.

Complex carbohydrates are in a lot of foods, but the highest levels of complex carbs are found in foods like bread, pasta, rice, cereal, and potatoes. Each serving of one of these carb-loaded foods provides 30–40 grams of carbs per 1 cup or 2 slices of bread. Now, let's just say you have 1–2 servings of these foods at each meal, which brings your carb total to 120–240 grams of carbs. Take this number and compare it to the recommended daily carb intake for each calorie level.

CARBOHYDRATE RECOMMENDATIONS FOR YOUR CALORIE LEVEL

Calories	1,200	1,400	1,600	1,800	2,000	2,200	2,400
Carbohydrates (grams)	180	210	240	270	300	330	360
Calories	2,600	2,800	3,000	3,200	3,400	3,600	
Carbohydrates (grams)	390	420	450	480	510	540	

Note: Minimum carbohydrate intake per day should not drop below 120 grams.

That calculation does work, because you haven't included all the other sources of carbs in your diet. Beans, nuts, fruits, vegetables, and dairy contain carbs, too. Let's try this again, working backward. If you are on a 1,200-calorie diet, then the recommended carb intake is 180 grams of carbs per day. You need to aim for 7–11 servings per day of fruits and vegetables; this will provide approximately 65–100 grams of carbs. You also want to try for a daily serving of beans or lentils, which provides another 30–40 grams of carbs per day. Let's just assume you are a rock star and got in 11 servings of fruits and vegetables and your daily bean serving, which leaves you with only 40 grams of carbs for whole-grain starches and really nothing left over for any added sugars. That is really quite perfect. So, instead of trying for a low-carb diet, it's better to get the carbs you need from the right sources: fruits, vegetables, and beans.

No Carbs Stand Alone

Another solution for your blood sugar is to plan your meals carefully. If you eat a meal including complex carbs and fiber, paired with both protein and the right types of fats, your blood sugar will respond in a different, more desirable way. Eating a well-balanced meal will leave your blood sugar more stable, keep you feeling more satisfied, and ward off rebound hunger until your next meal or snack time. With your blood sugar in balance, your body will be running more smoothly, reducing the amounts of insulin secreted while lowering both triglycerides and cholesterol. Win-win!

CHAPTER 2

The Big Essentials: Fiber, Water, and Fat

The foundation of the blood sugar diet is to transform your current nutritional routine into a high-fiber diet with adequate protein and moderate amounts of healthy fats. Balancing each essential ingredient in this diet is key to maintaining a desirable blood sugar level with very few fluctuations after a meal. Eating in this way will help you achieve and maintain a healthy weight while reducing your risk of diabetes, and will also give you tons of energy.

The Unbelievable Benefits of Fiber

Where does fiber fit into a healthy diet? Fiber really doesn't "fit in"; it is actually the star of the show when it comes to blood sugar control. Fiber is a type of complex carb that slows down the process of digestion and absorption, which plays a critical role in weight management and blood sugar stability. Diets containing adequate amounts of fiber are directly linked with weight loss success due to its ability to make you feel full.

Think of a balloon blowing up in your stomach. When you eat foods that contain fiber, the fiber absorbs water and expands in your stomach to make you feel full. This process helps you feel satisfied and helps you to stop eating, which will reduce your calorie intake and help you lose weight. Meals containing a combination of foods including complex carbohydrates and fiber slow digestion and absorption of sugar in your bloodstream, resulting in gradual changes in blood sugar, which is an excellent way to control or prevent diabetes and other diseases.

In addition to weight loss and blood sugar control, eating a variety of foods that contain fiber will help your body enjoy the additional benefits of fiber. There are two types of fiber: soluble and insoluble. The soluble type is the fiber that helps lower your cholesterol. This fiber acts like a sponge and soaks up circulating cholesterol, then transports it out of your body. This is an important process, because your body is trained to recycle the cholesterol. Therefore, this is one of the only ways to get extra cholesterol out of your body. The second type of fiber is insoluble, which helps keep you regular. Not only will this type of fiber help you use the bathroom without problems, but it also helps keep your colon healthy. The good news is that most foods with fiber contain a blend of the two types, which is beneficial for your body.

FACT

The average American eats only 15 grams of fiber per day. This doesn't even meet the recommended fiber intake for toddlers! First, it is important to identify your minimum fiber requirement for the day. Then you can work to increase it.

Fitting in Fiber

Fiber gets its name from the fibrous materials in our foods like seeds, skins, and even the little stringy parts of the orange. Foods with whole grains, such as cereals, breads, tortillas, and pastas can be good sources of fiber, provided there are more than 3 grams of fiber per serving. Fruits and vegetables have thick skins, seeds, and other fibrous materials that make them a great choice as well, containing on average 1–4 grams of fiber per serving or per piece of fruit. But the high-fiber award goes to legumes such as beans and lentils, giving you a whopping 8–16 grams of fiber per cup.

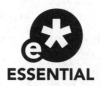

ESSENTIAL

Some favorite high-fiber grain brands include Oroweat, Kashi, All-Bran, Fiber One, Quaker, La Tortilla Factory, and Bob's Red Mill. Be sure to read the labels; not all of the products are high in fiber.

DAILY GRAMS OF FIBER REQUIRED BY GENDER AND AGE		
Age	**Females**	**Males**
1–3 years	19	19
4–8 years	25	25
9–13 years	26	31
14–18 years	26	38
19–30 years	25	38
31–50 years	25	38
51–70 years	21	30
70+ years	21	30

Take a minute to see how you are doing in terms of fiber intake. Look at the food you eat in one day, counting up the grams of fiber, and then compare it to your goal. You will get there by eating 7–11 servings of fruits and vegetables, 1–2 servings of beans, and a few whole grains.

FACT

Fiber is an important part of your diet. If you doubled your fiber, you could cut 100 calories from your daily diet. This means you'd lose 10 pounds per year.

Here are some simple ways to maximize your fiber intake:

- Choose high-fiber breakfast cereals and breads (at least 3 grams of fiber per serving). It helps if you look for the key word *bran*.
- Add 1–2 tablespoons ground flaxseed or 1 tablespoon chia seeds to hot cereals or yogurt (adds 2–5 grams of fiber).
- Choose your bread carefully. Good choices include breads with a lot of grainy pieces, whole-grain or stone-ground varieties, and sourdough. The goal is to choose bread that has more than 3 grams of fiber per slice and is made of whole grains.
- Eat fresh fruits instead of drinking fruit juices.
- Choose whole-grain pastas and brown rice.
- Increase your vegetable intake, including a variety of beans.
- Eat the skins of potatoes.
- Enjoy fresh fruits and vegetables in place of the common convenient snack foods.

In general, foods without labels, such as fruits and vegetables, should automatically go in your shopping cart, but when looking at foods with labels, use this guide to decide if the food is coming with you or staying put on the shelf. For foods with labels, keep an eye out for their fiber claims. In order to make a claim about the fiber content, the manufacturer must abide by labeling laws, which require:

- "Whole-grain" products to contain 100 percent whole-wheat flour
- "High-fiber" products to contain 5 grams of fiber or more per serving
- Products labeled "good source of fiber" to contain 2.4–4.9 grams of fiber per serving

When reading the label, direct your eyes straight to the fiber, then peek a little higher to compare it to the total carbohydrates. The closer these numbers are, the better. For example, find the label (either online, *www.latortillafactory.com/view/products/low-carb-high-fiber-tortillas*, or in-store) for the Low Carb, High Fiber Traditional Flour Tortillas made by La Tortilla Factory to practice.

Each tortilla contains 9 grams of fiber and 15 grams of total carbohydrates. Compared with the average tortilla, which contains 1–2 grams of fiber and 25 grams of carbs, this low-carb, high-fiber tortilla is a great choice. As you get more practice looking at food labels you will get a better sense of which foods are good sources of fiber and which are not. Don't forget to check the serving size. This doesn't mean you have to eat this serving size, but it's important to know how much food the nutrition label is talking about.

ALERT

A note of caution! When increasing fiber, you should increase your water intake, too. Otherwise your stomach will be very uncomfortable and you may find yourself spending way too long *waiting* in the bathroom.

What about Water?

Most people are walking around chronically dehydrated, falling well short of their daily fluid goals, unintentionally slowing their metabolic rates. This obviously can't be good, as water is essential for your metabolism, not to mention staying alive. Hydration directly affects your blood sugar: If you are dehydrated, your blood and blood sugar are more concentrated.

FACT

Thirst is often mistaken for hunger. Drinking two glasses of water before a meal has been shown to help reduce calorie intake. Order a glass of water before ordering anything else when out to eat.

The common water recommendation is eight (8-fluid-ounce) glasses a day, but this is not accurate for everyone. Water needs are more individualized depending on your weight, activity level, state of health, and the climate where you live. The Academy of Nutrition and Dietetics recommends drinking 9 cups (72 fluid ounces) water per day for women and 13 cups (104 fluid ounces) water per day for men.

QUESTION

How do you calculate water needs using your weight?
Another rule of thumb is to take your weight in pounds and divide it in half to calculate your goal water intake. For example, if you weigh 150 pounds, you require about 75 fluid ounces water per day.

Once you figure out how much water you need a day, consider that you should aim to drink 80 percent of your fluid intake. You can count all of the fluids you consume toward your fluid goal. Be aware that you should limit the amounts of caffeinated beverages and alcohol you are counting, as both of these in excess will lead to dehydration. Ideally, water should be your fluid of choice. If you choose another beverage, be sure to check the label. Beverages may contain excessive calories, added sugar, caffeine, and alcohol, all which need to be considered before you make the choice to drink them. There is a time and a place for drinks like Gatorade, Powerade, and coconut water; most people doing casual exercise do not need this level of rehydration.

FACT

On any given day, the average person loses about 2½ quarts (80 ounces) of water. This doesn't even take into consideration whether it is hot or humid out. Remember to replace this water. Check the color when you use the restroom; your urine should be pale if you are doing your job!

The remaining 20 percent of your water intake will come from the food you eat. Foods that contain a great amount of water and fiber slow down the digestion process, leaving you feeling fuller longer. Water-filled foods like fruits and vegetables are most often extremely healthy choices that provide you with a multitude of additional health benefits.

Although you can't meet 100 percent of your fluid needs from foods alone, you can make the most of the foods you choose. Here is a list of the best water-loaded foods:

- More than 90 percent water: watermelon, cabbage, celery, spinach, cauliflower, zucchini, lettuce, tomato, broccoli, strawberries, grapefruit, cantaloupe, peppers, cucumbers, eggplant
- More than 75 percent water: pineapple, apples, oranges, carrots, pear, peach, plums, blueberries, raspberries, grapes

Anytime you sweat, whether it is through exercise or just because it's hot outside, you need to drink some additional water to replace the fluids you've lost. Try drinking 5–8 ounces water for every 20 minutes of exercise or heat exposure.

Maximize the H_2O

Water is essential to keep you alive. In fact, you would only survive approximately one week without it! Other than the obvious function of hydration, water also plays the important role of removing toxins from your body and is a key component in energy metabolism (weight management) in your body. Here are some tips to maximize the metabolic rate of your water intake:

- Drink water prior to each meal and throughout the day.
- Drink water prior to the start of your outdoor activities.
- Always bring a water bottle with you when you leave the house.
- If drinking alcohol, alternate each alcoholic beverage with a full glass of water.
- Keep a glass or bottle of water at your desk, and you will drink more water without even trying.
- Instead of a coffee or snack break, take a water break.

- Instead of an alcoholic beverage or soda, drink sparkling water at your next party.
- Divide up your water needs and set goals throughout the day (e.g., drink 30 ounces of water by noon).

Fat Essentials

There are quite a few misconceptions when it comes to fat in your diet. Some people think you need it, while others avoid fat like the plague. The fact is your body requires some fat from your diet. Not only is the amount of fat you eat important, but the type of fat is important, too.

A few things to remember about fat:

- Too much fat results in fat storage (weight gain).
- Fat provides your body with energy. It provides 9 calories per gram, more than double the amount of calories from carbs or protein!
- Fats take longer to break down during digestion; therefore, they help satisfy hunger and help regulate blood sugar.

Fat can be broken up into a few groups based on the structures, but to keep things simple, let's divide fats into the good, plant-based fats and the not-so-good fats that are animal-based.

Monounsaturated and polyunsaturated fats are the preferred fats, as they are the heart-healthy fats that come from plant sources such as olive, sunflower, and safflower oils, avocado, and nuts. A diet based around these fats can lower your LDL ("bad") cholesterol. Of these heart-healthy fats, there are two types that are considered essential. Your body is unable to produce these; therefore, you must include these foods in your diet daily to meet your needs.

The essential fatty acids (EFAs) include alpha-linolenic acid (omega-3) and linoleic acid (omega-6). The current American diet consists of a ratio of these two fats of 10:1 to 25:1 omega-6:omega-3, but the desirable goal is 4:1, or, even better, 1:1! The balance of omega-6 and omega-3 is essential for optimal metabolism and weight loss. Adequate amounts of EFAs help reduce the risk of heart disease by preventing clogging of the arteries. Good sources of EFAs are olive oil, canola oil, flaxseed, flaxseed oil, nuts, avocado, and fish.

FACT

According to the Centers for Disease Control, excessive intake of saturated fat, trans fat, and cholesterol in the diet can lead to weight gain and increase your risk of several life-threatening diseases, including four of the top seven causes of death in the United States.

Animal sources provide the majority of saturated fat in the American diet. It is important to limit your intake of saturated fat to 7 percent total calories per day due to its ability to increase your blood cholesterol levels and increase your risk of heart disease. Foods high in saturated fats include whole-fat dairy (whole milk, cheese, ice cream, 2% milk, sour cream, cream cheese), high-fat meats (regular ground beef, hot dogs, sausages, bologna, bacon, and ribs), poultry (skin or darker meat), condiments (butter, lard, cream sauces, gravy), and oils (palm).

Eating animal products provides the body with not only saturated fats but also cholesterol. Your body actually makes enough cholesterol to perform its roles in the body; that extra dietary cholesterol is not a necessity. Therefore, it is important to limit your dietary cholesterol to 300 milligrams per day, maybe even less—closer to 200 milligrams per day if you have any risk of diabetes or heart disease. Intake exceeding the recommended amount may result in an increased blood cholesterol level and increased risk of heart disease. Foods high in cholesterol include organ meats (animal brain and liver), eggs, shrimp, high-fat dairy foods, high-fat meat, and poultry skin.

Another one of the bad types of fat is trans fat. This is the worst type of fat for your heart. It increases your cholesterol and your risk of heart disease. This type of fat is formed when liquid oils are hydrogenated (changed) and made into a solid fat, which is done to allow foods to be kept longer on the shelf. Trans fats are often found in vegetable shortenings, some stick margarines, shelf-stable snack foods, foods made with partially hydrogenated oils such as baked goods, and foods fried in partially hydrogenated oils such as French fries.

Trans fats are now easy to identify because of the new labeling law requiring trans fats to be included on the nutrition facts label. The American Heart Association recommends limiting trans fats to less than 1 percent of your daily total calories. Try limiting to less than 2 grams per day. Foods that contain 0.5 grams trans fats or less may claim 0 grams trans fats per serving, so you could easily exceed this recommendation without even knowing it. So, in order to avoid trans fats as much as possible, scan the list of ingredients for the word "hydrogenated"—for example, "partially hydrogenated soybean oil"—and skip these foods.

How Much Fat Won't Make You Fat?

The recommendations from the American Heart Association are to limit the calories from fat to less than 30 percent per day. If you have a risk of heart disease (family history, high blood pressure, high cholesterol, overweight, and/or diabetes), you may want to consider limiting to 20 percent calories from fat per day. Your saturated fat intake should be less than 7 percent calories per day or ¼ of your fat intake. Here is a guide on how to apply the recommendations:

ESTIMATED FAT REQUIREMENTS							
Calories	**1,200**	**1,400**	**1,600**	**1,800**	**2,000**	**2,200**	
30% fat (grams)	40	47	53	60	67	73	
20% fat (grams)	27	31	36	40	44	49	
Saturated fat (grams)	9	11	12	14	16	17	
Trans fat (grams)	1.25	1.5	1.75	2	2.25	2.5	
Calories	**2,400**	**2,600**	**2,800**	**3,000**	**3,200**	**3,400**	**3,600**
30% fat (grams)	80	87	93	100	107	113	120
20% fat (grams)	53	58	62	67	71	76	80
Saturated fat (grams)	19	20	22	23	25	26	28
Trans fat (grams)	2.75	3	3.25	3.5	3.75	4	4.25

1. Multiply the calories from fat by 3. The answer must be less than the total calories per serving to be less than 30 percent. For example, if there are 100 calories from fat, you multiply by 3 to get 300. This number is greater than the total calories (230); therefore, this food does not meet the goal of 30 percent or less calories from fat.
2. Check the percent daily value for saturated fat. This number should be less than 7 percent. For example, if the food label states 10 percent of the daily value for saturated fat, which is greater than your goal of less than 7 percent desired value of saturated fat; therefore, this food does not meet the goal of 7 percent calories from saturated fat or less.
3. Look for foods that have 0 grams trans fat and 0 milligrams cholesterol. Your goal is to keep trans fat as low as possible and keep cholesterol less than 200 milligrams per day.

Cut the Fat

Excessive fat can be lurking where you least expect it. Here are some tips to help identify and cut out the extra (unhealthy) fats:

1. Eat fewer fried foods; try for a goal of 1–2 times per month, max. Foods to limit/avoid: French fries, grilled sandwiches, hash browns, deep-fried foods, fried chicken, refried beans, tempura, doughnuts, chips, corn dogs, onion rings. Better choices: fresh fruits, raw vegetables, baked potato, angel food cake, low-fat crackers, boiled beans.
2. Use less fat when cooking. Ingredients to avoid when cooking: butter, lard, margarine, bacon grease, mayonnaise, creamy salad dressing. Ways to prepare foods with less fat: broil, bake, barbecue, boil, steam, microwave, and use cooking spray in place of extra butter or oils.
3. Eat fewer high-fat foods. Foods to limit/avoid: bacon, sausage, pepperoni, ribs, chicken wings, hamburgers, hot dogs, salami, pastrami, cookies, pastries, whole-fat dairy products such as whole or 2% milk, cheeses, cream cheese, half-and-half, cream, creamed soups, peanut butter, nuts, chocolate. Better choices: low-fat mayonnaise or salad dressing, chicken or turkey without skin, low-fat deli meats, ground beef (90–96% lean), egg substitutes, beans, nonfat or 1% milk, low-fat yogurt, low-fat cheeses.

ESSENTIAL

Know the facts when reading labels with claims regarding their fat content. If a product is labeled "light," that tells you that it has ⅓ less calories or 50 percent less fat than the regular product. A "reduced-fat" product has 25 percent less fat than the regular product. A "fat-free" food has less than 0.5 grams of fat, while a "low-fat" food has 3 grams or less of fat.

The Pros and Fats of Fish

Fish are one of nature's best sources of omega-3 fatty acids, which have positive effects on heart health. Omega-3 fatty acids have been found to lower blood pressure, lower heart rate, prevent arteries from hardening, lower triglycerides, and reduce the risk of heart disease, the leading cause of death for all men and women in the world. The American Heart Association recommends eating fish two times per week. Intake of fish also has been associated with decreases in mental decline with age and decreased risk of depression.

Fish is also a good source of protein, vitamins including niacin, B_6, B_{12}, vitamin A, and vitamin D, and minerals including iron, phosphorus, iodine, and selenium. Fish is also low in saturated fat and cholesterol, with the exceptions of shrimp and crab.

The fish with the highest amounts of omega-3 fatty acids are:

- Fresh tuna
- Herring
- Mackerel
- Lake trout
- Salmon
- Sole
- Halibut

Some fish contain mercury, but it is unclear if this has bad effects on health for men and women. Pregnant women are advised to avoid the four types of fish with the highest mercury content: shark, swordfish, mackerel, and bass. Other fish should still be consumed in moderation to provide adequate omega-3 fatty acids for brain development of the infant.

Enjoy fish two times per week as part of a heart-healthy diet. If fish is not a part of your diet, be sure to get your omega-3 fatty acids in other foods, including olive oil, soybean oil, walnut oil, and flaxseed oil.

The Power of Proteins

Last but certainly not least is protein. Most people are so concerned with making sure they are getting enough protein in their diet that they often overdo it. The reality is that protein is essential, but your body really doesn't need as much as you may think. You can easily achieve your protein requirements if you focus on protein-rich plant sources, including fiber-rich beans and lentils.

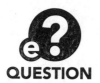

QUESTION

How much protein do you really need?
Grab your calculator and figure out your protein needs. Take your body weight in pounds and multiply it by 0.4 to get the grams of protein required per day. For example, if your weight is 160 pounds, multiply by 0.4 to get your protein needs of 64 grams per day.

Proteins are made up of chains of amino acids, nine of which are considered essential to your body. You have to get these essential amino acids from your diet because the body can't make them. The other amino acids are considered nonessential due to the body's ability to make them.

Protein has many important roles in the body:

- Involved in muscle contractions—think about the heart muscle!
- Helps regulate water balance—think about the kidneys and hydration
- Makes hormones, enzymes, and other body components important in metabolism
- Provides energy when carbohydrates and fats are not available
- Bonus: Foods high in protein also provide iron, B vitamins, and minerals
- Another bonus: Foods high in protein don't increase your blood sugar

In order for your body to make proteins to complete all of the functions, you must get adequate amounts of essential amino acids in your diet. Chances are that you are getting adequate amounts of protein with your current diet. It would be ideal to transition your protein intake to more vegetarian sources, including beans, lentils, nuts, and whole grains. Even though the proteins from vegetarian sources are considered incomplete proteins (not containing all the essential amino acids), if you eat a good variety of these foods throughout the day, you will be able to meet your essential amino acid needs. (See Appendix B for high-fiber and high-protein choices.) Fish is also a great source of protein; every ounce of fish provides 7 grams of protein. Each serving of the recipes in Chapter 13: Flavorful Fish provides 28 grams of protein.

CHAPTER 3

Your Guide to Building and Balancing Your Meals

Grocery shopping, meal planning, and preparing breakfast, lunch, and dinner may seem overwhelming and time-consuming. Don't worry. If you take each task step by step, you will see that following the blood sugar diet isn't as difficult as you would expect. In fact, this lifestyle is completely maintainable. The key to success is stocking your kitchen with the right foods, including meals that can be whipped up in minutes on your busy weeknights.

Grocery Shopping with a Plan of Attack

There are a few important measures to take before heading to your grocery store. First, be sure to do your homework. This includes reading the store ads, if you have time, to see what is on sale. Sale items can inspire your weekly menu and keep you from getting into a boring rut. The second step is to be sure you are ready to shop, specifically that you are not hungry. If you are full, then you will be less likely to surrender to the temptations of poor food choices and impulse buys.

Once you enter the store, head straight to the produce section. This is where the majority of your cart should be filled. Your goal is to eat 7–11 servings of fruits and vegetables per day, so if you are buying food for the week, you will need to buy approximately 49–77 servings of fruits and vegetables for each person in your house. Stock up on a variety of the seasonal fruits and vegetables. You can usually identify the seasonal foods by the sale items, but also check out Appendix C for a seasonal guide. You may also want to visit a local famers' market to stock up on fresh seasonal fruits and vegetables. Try to keep an open mind when it comes to trying new foods like spaghetti squash, eggplant, asparagus, Brussels sprouts, sweet potatoes, papaya, mango, and kiwi, all rich in vitamins, minerals, fiber, and antioxidants.

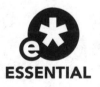

ESSENTIAL

Try buying wholesale. Since your goal is to shoot for 49–77 servings of vegetables and fruits per person in your household per week, you may try purchasing larger packages of produce for a reduced price. This may make you feel overwhelmed due to the enormous size of the packages, but you can do it if you take on the challenge to finish the produce before it goes bad.

Once you have made your rounds in the produce section, take a trip to the bean aisle. Grab a few bags of high-fiber and high-protein dried beans and lentils; these will take a bit more time but not much effort to prepare. You may also want to grab a few cans of beans, black-eyed peas, and chick-peas to drain, rinse, and use on nights when you are short on time. For additional protein, take your cart for a drive through the nut section; grab a bag or two of pistachios, almonds, or walnuts, and a jar of almond butter. Lastly, grab yourself at least two servings of omega-3-fatty-acid-rich fish such as tilapia, trout, or salmon.

FACT

Dried beans are great for your budget when compared to canned beans. You get 8 cups of prepared dried beans for every 2 cups of canned beans. This doesn't mean you have to do all dried beans—canned beans can be rinsed and used when you're in a rush.

While you are in the canned foods aisle, think about grabbing a can or two of your favorite vegetables. These can be rinsed to reduce the sodium content and cooked up quickly on busy nights. You may also want to grab a jar of olives, sun-dried tomatoes, and pepperoncini to help add flavor to your foods, especially your salads. As you continue through the processed foods aisles (anything that has a label), be prepared to read between the lines. The nutrition facts label is full of information; the trick is in knowing where to look to find it and then understanding what it means. The grocery store can be a busy place, so it is essential to flip that package and evaluate it in ten seconds or less, because who has the extra time to spend in the grocery store?

Depending on the food choice, look at the label for specific things. When you hit the bread and cereal aisle, review the label specifically for fiber. Be sure you get at least 3 grams of fiber per serving. Oatmeal is another great choice; consider trying the steel-cut variety as the oats are less processed, and therefore take longer to break down, resulting in slower changes in blood sugar, which keeps you satisfied longer. Grab a bag of ground flaxseed, chia seeds, or shelled hemp seeds; these are all great choices of the essential fats, so no need to check these labels. If you find yourself in the frozen food aisle, take advantage and stock up on bags of frozen vegetables and fruits, especially the ones that are not in season. If you feel that you need an ultra-quick meal, check the frozen meals aisle for one that fits the bill: at least 3 grams of fiber, less than 500 milligrams of sodium, and 500 calories or fewer. Plan on adding fresh vegetables to this meal to make it more satisfying. Try to steer clear of the frozen pizzas, ice cream, and other desserts. Save these treats for special occasions outside the house.

For dairy and dairy replacements, be sure to read the label for the saturated fat content and make sure the one you choose has at least 30 percent of the daily value for calcium per serving. While you are in the neighborhood, you may want to pick up a container of Smart Balance, which is a blend of healthy unsaturated fats without cholesterol, a way better choice than butter.

Before getting in the checkout line, give your cart a once-over to be sure your purchases are as colorful as you want your plate to be.

Stretch your dollar by stocking up on some thrifty foods, including dry beans, oatmeal, sweet potatoes, spinach, frozen vegetables, whole-grain rice, frozen fruits, onions, and peppers. These staples can be used to make so many recipes and smoothies.

Meal Planning with Color

Meal planning sounds as if it may take a lot of time and preparation, and let's be honest, who has that kind of time? Realistic meal planning involves opening the refrigerator and trying to figure out what you can throw together with the little time you have. A quick way to ensure that you are planning a balanced meal is to use the colors of your foods as your guide. Think of your plate as a blank canvas—the more colors you add, the better your nutrition masterpiece will turn out.

First, envision a common meal, such as chicken, mashed potatoes and gravy, and corn. This meal is all the different shades of boring. Now take similar ingredients and transform this blah meal into a masterpiece. Start with a bed of vibrant green spinach, layer on small slivers of grilled chicken, roasted corn, and chopped red peppers, and serve with a baked sweet potato and a small bowl full of blueberries. Now that is a colorful meal! Not only do the added colors bring visual appeal to the meal, but they also bring large amounts of fiber and antioxidants to improve the taste bud appeal.

If your usual meal-planning instincts lead you more toward the meat-and-potato type of meal, then it is time to try switching things up with this new approach. The first step in planning is reversing your mindset: Start by choosing your vegetables and save the meat and potatoes for last (if they fit in at all). By choosing vegetables first, your meal is more likely to be fiber focused and your plate will be colorful. Ideally, you have taken full advantage of the produce in season and stocked your refrigerator with a variety of veggies. Look through your crisper and see what you have to work with, and then get creative. If you have green onions, cilantro, bok choy, spinach, broccoli, and mushrooms, this may make a great start to a soup. Or if you find bell peppers, zucchini, red onions, mushrooms, carrots, and cabbage, these could be stir-fried together with olive oil. Give your onions, green beans, broccoli, carrots, or Brussels sprouts a quick slicing, toss with olive oil, and roast them in the oven for a quick side dish with unbelievable flavor and very little effort. If you have only spinach and broccoli in the refrigerator, make the most of it by sautéing these two with chopped garlic in olive oil for another quick and powerful green side to your dinner.

The great thing about starting out your meal with vegetables is that you can be generous with the portions in order to get your 7–11 servings (including fruits) per day. Try filling at least half your plate with vegetables. Additional vegetable servings provide far more benefits than harm! The usual portion size for vegetables and fruits is 1 cup raw, ½ cup cooked, or 1 medium fruit.

ESSENTIAL

The goal is to always have a few go-to veggie recipes that you enjoy and that take very little prep time, such as oven-roasted green beans and boiled corn on the cob. But, if you are completely rushed for time, try serving edamame, frozen vegetables, or baby carrots to add color to your time-sensitive meal.

Your next step should be to choose your protein source, ideally a plant-based protein such as beans, lentils, or legumes. If meat is part of your everyday routine, be sure to choose meats that are low in saturated fat, such as fish, chicken breast, 94% lean ground beef, and pork chops. Make an effort to serve more meatless meals than meat-containing meals throughout the week. This can be achieved by branching out of your recipe repertoire to include new recipes with all types of beans and lentils. These protein sources may be incorporated into your vegetable dish or served on their own. Chickpeas, black beans, and pinto beans go well in a veggie stir-fry, lentils and vegetables combine to make a great stew, and, of course, all of the above can be added to a spinach salad.

The usual portion size for meat, chicken, and fish is 3 ounces, which is the size of a deck of cards. A standard serving of beans is ½ cup, about half the size of your fist. Typically, the American diet is heavily focused on protein, usually exceeding what our bodies need. Although protein is essential for the body, excessive amounts may be stored as fat. Go ahead and try a few meals without the meat; your body won't miss it a bit.

Beans, lentils, and legumes actually serve a dual purpose, providing both protein and fiber. But if you feel the need to add a complex carb to your meal, make sure to choose fiber-rich whole-grain breads and pastas, brown rice, or sweet potatoes. The serving size for this category is one slice of bread, one small to medium sweet potato with skin, or ½ cup pasta, rice, beans, lentils, or legumes. Similar to your protein servings, grains are often overserved, which will lead to additional fat storage as well.

Fat plays an important role in your body. Most people instinctively feel the need to limit all fat, but in actuality, a small amount of the healthier fats is essential to your metabolism. When planning your meal, choose the right fat in the right amount. A couple safe fats to stock in your home are plant-based fats such as olive, canola, and soy oils, avocados, nuts and nut butters, ground flaxseed, and shelled hemp seed. The proper portion size for these fats is 1 teaspoon of oil, about the size of the tip of your thumb, or 1 ounce of avocado, about ⅕ of a medium avocado, and 1 ounce of nuts, less than a small handful. If your protein source is fish or nuts, you can count that toward both protein and healthy fat servings.

Of course, let's not forget the fruit! Fruit serves as the perfect sweet treat to top off a meal, and a single piece of fruit alone can help keep your appetite in control between mealtimes. Fruit is a much healthier alternative to any other dessert, especially in terms of your blood sugar control.

One last consideration for your meal planning is calcium. It is recommended that you have a minimum of three servings of dairy per day. This recommendation has been made for years, primarily to meet calcium requirements. If this is difficult for you to achieve, try to meet your calcium needs with alternative ways, including dark leafy green vegetables (collard greens, broccoli, kale, bok choy, edamame, and okra) and nondairy, calcium-rich milk alternatives. The good choices will have a label that reads 30–45 percent daily value for calcium; that's equivalent to a glass of low-fat milk. Dairy-free yogurts are also great choices for calcium and vitamin D.

Working Through the Weeknight Runaround

Weeknights can be the most hectic time to squeeze in a healthy meal. This is probably when you start thinking about ordering takeout or running to the drive-through. Your goal of whipping up a wholesome meal to nourish yourself and your loved ones may fall to the wayside when you are busy. The home option is obviously the healthier choice, but the reality is that the latest statistics from the U.S. Department of Agriculture say that most families are eating half to two-thirds of their meals outside of the home during the school year. This means you need to capitalize on the one meal you have complete control of: dinner. When it comes to the weeknight runaround there are a few ideas to make getting dinner on the table an easier assignment.

Tips for Success Monday Through Friday

1. **Start with a plan.** Write down all of your evening commitments in order to identify which nights you will have time to prepare a 30–45-minute meal and which nights will require a quick bite due to time constraints. Then plan your meal ideas for the week.
2. **Use your weekends wisely.** Weekends are a great time to get to the grocery store to stock up for the coming week's meals. When you buy fruits or vegetables, be sure to take the time to cut them up for meals or snacks. This will help save time during the week and also keep your produce from going bad.
3. **Get the family involved.** Making dinner should be a family affair. Allow the family to help set the table, mix ingredients, prepare simple foods, etc.
4. **Makeover your leftovers.** Cooking extra portions can be a timesaver for the following night. For example, always make an extra cup or two of beans, as they can be used in a variety of meals.

5. **Make the most of your time.** If time is limited, prepare one of these meals that are ready in 10 minutes or less:
   - **Grilled tomato and cheese sandwich:** Spray high-fiber bread (such as Oroweat Healthful Flax and Sunflower, Double Fiber, or Healthy Multi-Grain breads) with cooking spray or calorie-free butter spray, and top with low-fat or 2% cheese, tomatoes, and spinach. Serve with steamed broccoli or asparagus.
   - **Tuna melt:** Toast a high-fiber English muffin and top with tuna salad, tomato, and lettuce. Top with a sprinkle of shredded Cheddar cheese and place under broiler for 1–2 minutes. Serve with baby carrots, celery, and a bowl of strawberries and blueberries.
   - **Black bean taco wrap:** Take a high-fiber tortilla (such as La Tortilla Factory's Low Carb, High Fiber Traditional Flour Tortillas) and add drained, rinsed black beans, lettuce, tomato, low-fat shredded cheese, avocado slices, and salsa.
   - **Greek wrap:** Use romaine hearts as the wrap and layer with hummus, red pepper slices, tomato, cucumber slices, and kalamata olives.
   - **Quesadilla:** Spray a high-fiber tortilla with cooking spray, lay in skillet over medium-low heat, and top with drained, rinsed black beans, salsa, corn, spinach, onion, and a sprinkle of 2% pepper jack cheese. Once heated, fold in half and cut into triangles. Serve with a slice of avocado.
   - **Egg white or Egg Beaters scramble:** In a medium skillet, scramble egg white over medium heat until fluffy and cooked through. Add red peppers, spinach, onions, and mushrooms, and sprinkle with reduced-fat feta cheese; continue heating until hot. Serve with a variety of sliced fruits.
   - **Homemade rice bowl:** Layer rice, beans, tomatoes, lettuce, corn, and salsa in a bowl. Top with avocado or guacamole and a dollop of non-fat Greek yogurt.
   - **Sweet potatoes and salad:** Slice sweet potatoes into coins, place them in a single layer on a baking sheet, and broil for 5–10 minutes until soft and brown. Serve with a salad topped with olive oil dressing and a side of mango and strawberries topped with a drizzle of honey and cinnamon.
6. **Make your lunches the night before:**

- Top a whole-grain English muffin with hummus, spinach, avocado, and tomato. Have a side of sliced strawberries to round out the meal.
- Combine chickpeas, lettuce, tomato, and cheese in a high-fiber tortilla or on high-fiber bread. Serve with mashed avocado and homemade cinnamon applesauce.
- Portion carrots, red pepper, and cucumber slices for dipping in your homemade dressing and serve with a baked sweet potato and a fruit or vegetable smoothie.
- Prepare a green salad topped with walnuts, red onion, diced pears, and balsamic vinaigrette. Serve with a bowl of watermelon.

Meal Frequency

You may find yourself falling into some unhealthy routines. Maybe you skip breakfast one day because of the morning rush or you skip lunch because you didn't have time to pack one. The goal is to eat five to six times a day and avoid skipping meals. Most often when you skip a meal, you will overeat or splurge at the next meal.

Also when you routinely skip meals, your body and its metabolism may become confused. Going extended periods of time without food—for example, skipping breakfast—puts you in a fasting state for at least sixteen hours. At this point, your body will go into starvation and conservation mode and will ration the energy it expends (calories burned) because it is unsure when it will be fed again, and will package up any extra fuel to store as fat for later use (when another meal is skipped). These changes in your eating patterns will also lead to negative influences on your blood sugar.

In order to prevent this from happening, it is best to keep healthy snacks and meals available for emergency use. When you are faced with hunger and you have no food available, your healthy food options are few and far between. Most likely you will resort to fast foods or vending machine snacks, which are high in calories and fat.

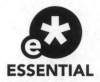
Portions in Proportion

Keeping portions in check is the key component to keeping your intake in balance in order to prevent fat storage. For example, one large orange may actually be 1½ servings of fruit due to its size. This is okay as long as you are aware and take portion sizes into account when planning your day. Even healthy foods can be consumed in excess amounts. The key is to keep your serving size appropriate to avoid excessive intake of nutrients. The absolute moral of the story is that excessive intake of fat, protein, and/or carbohydrates leads to storage of fat. Your body has requirements for each nutrient, but when consumed in excess, your body's "backup plan" is to send it to be packaged as fat to be used later.

Here are a few handy tips to help estimate your portions:

- 3 ounces meat, poultry, or fish = a deck of cards or the palm of a woman's hand
- 3 ounces fish = the size of your checkbook
- ½ cup fruit, vegetable, pasta, or rice = size of a small fist

- 1 ounce cheese = size of your thumb
- 1 tablespoon peanut butter = make a circle by touching thumb and first finger
- 1 serving fruit = size of a small fist

Check your portions. First serve your plate with your usual amounts of food and then use a measuring cup to see how big your serving actually is. You may be surprised that the serving is bigger or smaller than you thought!

Another way to keep portions in the right proportion to control your second helpings. When you head back to the kitchen for just a little bit more of your dinner, your best bet is to choose extra servings of vegetables. Typically the vegetables are going to be the lowest-calorie choice, as well as the most filling.

CHAPTER 4

Lifestyle Transition Guide

Making a lifestyle change involves taking a step back and evaluating all of the choices you are making in your day-to-day life. When it comes to healthy eating, planning ahead will maximize your success in all sorts of common situations that come your way. Before you go out to eat with friends or attend a holiday celebration, plan your strategy to make the best of each situation. This may consist of looking at the restaurant menu online, bringing a healthy dish, or identifying the best options and monitoring your portion sizes. Try to keep the focus on socializing and enjoying your life.

Changing Your Mindset

At first, it may seem like a stretch for you to take on this new lifestyle. Keep in mind that the ultimate goal of this change is blood sugar regulation. It is important for you to keep everything in perspective, and understand that this is truly a lifestyle and mindset change. The goal is to follow the blood sugar diet at least 80 percent of the time. Be sure to choose carefully and enjoy the 20 percent of the time that you decide to stray just a bit. These occasions need to be special, when you feel you really want/need to go for it. It may be best to just enjoy that cake at your friend's birthday party or your Thanksgiving dinner (within reason) and then just return back to the fundamentals of this diet.

You may be faced with temptation every day. Try to prepare yourself for the situations that may arise. Saying "no" to social opportunities that involve a splurge can be difficult, but most often you can make a healthy choice or simply and kindly turn down a dessert. Always carry healthy snacks with you to avoid making poor decisions out of hunger.

Making a decision happens in a split second, such as when the waitress arrives to take your order. If during that split second you can make the better choice, you will be very successful and much healthier as a result. Eventually, this will make these decisions easier on you as you get more momentum and feel your health improve.

Cleaning Out the Cupboards

One of the most important steps in successfully implementing the blood sugar diet is to make over your kitchen. Look closely at all of the items in your refrigerator and your pantry to evaluate whether they should stay or go. One of the quickest ways to nix the bad stuff would be to remove anything with sugar in the first three ingredients on the nutrition label. The items without labels are most likely the things you should buy more of.

Once you have cleansed your kitchen, stock it with a good variety of the staples and try your very hardest not to bring tempting and possibly blood sugar–spiking foods into your home. If there is something you would like to splurge on, try going out somewhere to get it. Avoid sabotaging your diet by buying your splurge at the grocery store and bringing it home, because usually these packaged items include several servings that will test your willpower.

ALERT

It may be difficult to know which packages you need to throw away. One way to evaluate an item's worth is to look at the ingredients. If there are words you don't know how to pronounce, pitch it. Exceptions may be frozen fruits, vegetables, and beans, but again be sure to read the label to confirm that is all that is really in there.

Here is a list of the staples to stock in your kitchen:

- Fresh, frozen, and canned vegetables
- Fresh and frozen fruits, especially avocado
- Dried, frozen, and canned beans, peas, lentils, and refrigerated hummus
- Variety of nuts
- High-fiber tortillas and cereals, brown rice, and sweet potatoes
- Fresh and frozen fish, lean meat, and poultry
- Ground flaxseed, shelled hemp seed, and olive oil

Dining Out with a Plan

Most popular fast-food restaurants have a value menu of some sort. On paper, it's an amazing deal. A hamburger, a side of fries, and a drink—all one dollar each. This is great for your wallet, but what about your waistline?

The Wendy's Right Price Right Size Menu has some delicious items, such as the Junior Bacon Cheeseburger, four-piece chicken nuggets, French fries, and chicken wraps, but there is an average of 46 percent calories from fat in these items! This is way too much, as your goal is to keep your foods under 30 percent calories from fat. So these one-dollar deals are not the best, but what can you order that won't put your heart and health in danger? The Grilled Chicken Wrap has the lowest percent of calories from fat at 36 percent. This would go nicely with a side salad, mandarin orange cup, or baked potato. These items would decrease the meal's fat composition to closer to 30 percent.

America's favorite fast-food chain, McDonald's, received the wrath of the media after the documentary *Super Size Me* came out in 2004, but they also responded with an attempt to make their menu items "healthier." But how did they do? They are using healthier oils, their foods are now trans fat–free, and they have added apple slices, yogurt parfaits, Go-Gurt, and salads to the menu, but what about the dollar menu? The menu contains a few sandwiches, the McDouble, Double Cheeseburger, and McChicken sandwich, which have 39–44 percent of calories from fat. Again, your goal is to keep your foods under 30 percent from fat. And don't forget the fries, another whopping 45 percent calories from fat!

Some of the more traditional family restaurants are trying to provide healthier alternatives as well, and some even include the nutrition information on the menu. If the meal is not marked as a healthier choice, review the description of the meal closely looking for red-flag words. These may include the obvious one, *fried*, but also *creamy, breaded, cream sauce, butter, mayo,* etc. Better choices are usually described as baked, broiled, grilled, or steamed. If you are unsure about your choice, ask the server. For example, do the steamed vegetables have butter added? Sometimes the things you may assume are healthy are not. Sushi and salads can be a great example of secret diet sabotage. Sushi may be supersized with extra rice and topped with calorie-rich sauces, and the same goes for the toppings and dressing on your salad. Try customizing your meal to meet your needs. Most restaurants will cater to whatever requests you have.

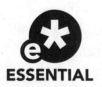

Here are some tips to help you enjoy your meal out of the house without any extra guilt:

- Try to be part of the decision of where to eat; that way, you can avoid all-you-can-eat buffets and other extremely unhealthy options.
- Check the restaurant menu and nutrition facts online and formulate your plan before you go out.
- Avoid arriving to the restaurant starving. This could cause you to eat excessive amounts, especially if you are at a restaurant that provides complimentary chips and salsa or bread and butter.
- Split an entrée with your friend.
- Pack up half of your meal to take home. If it sits on your plate, the temptation will eat at you for the whole meal, and it may even win.
- Always order the small option, such as the lunch portion, a half order, or the à la carte option if available.
- Order an appetizer as your meal; these are usually smaller portions that pair nicely with a side salad.
- Start with a glass of water and continue drinking water throughout the course of your meal. This will help fill you up, reducing how much you eat. Remember, you can always take your food home and enjoy it for another meal.
- Try a vegetable-rich meal such as a salad, and be sure to request the dressing on the side. If you have a choice in dressing, consider olive oil and vinegar or any other vinaigrette they offer.

Nutrition on the Road

If you are counting down the days to your next getaway, then now is the time to do your research on what you should and should not eat on the road. No matter your destination, try not to let your vacation be a free pass to indulge in high-calorie and high-fat foods. This type of eating will leave you with an unwanted souvenir around your waistline well after the vacation ends.

Before you leave, think about your travel plans. If you have a long flight, drive, or train ride, pack healthy snacks to munch on when you get hungry. Snack choices that are available when you are traveling usually consist of packaged food high in sodium and fat, not to mention the fact that highways and airports are packed with fast-food restaurants, which can easily find a way to pack 700–2,000 calories into one meal.

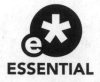

ESSENTIAL

Fuel up your car and your body at the gas station. The options are usually limited, but you may be able to score a piece of fresh fruit, a bag of mixed nuts or sunflower seeds, a nut-based bar, or air-popped popcorn.

Here are some tips to help you while on vacation:

- **Think about the plans you have for the day and bring some foods that will help prevent desperate eating.** Try to plan where and when you'll be eating so you can choose healthy restaurants. Here are some travel-friendly snack ideas that will help keep you on track:
  1. Carrots, celery, red pepper strips, and cherry tomatoes
  2. Baked sweet potato fries
  3. Edamame or chickpeas
  4. A mix of high-fiber cereal, nuts, and dried fruit
  5. Apples, pears, bananas, oranges, grapes, and peaches
  6. Ants on a log (celery topped with peanut butter and raisins)
  7. Granola bars
  8. Low-fat popcorn
  9. Sunflower seeds, pumpkin seeds, and almonds
- **Eating the local favorite foods should be part of your vacation, but make a plan to do so in moderation.** For example, one approach is to have two good, sound nutritious meals such as a continental breakfast of fruit and whole grains (possibly flaxseed if you brought it with you) and a great salad for lunch, then enjoy the local favorite for dinner.
- **Find the grocery store or farmers' market closest to your destination and buy fruits and veggies in bulk for the duration of your trip.** Just imagine all the calories and fat you will avoid by pairing your fast-food sandwich with carrots and strawberries instead of French fries. (You will save 130–400 calories every day, which will help prevent ¼–1 pound of weight gain over your 7–10-day vacation!)

- **Fruity poolside drinks, as well as other types of alcohol and mixed drinks, can provide quite a few calories.** Try drinking in moderation and alternating drinks with a glass of water to prevent dehydration.
- **Exercise should be a major part of your vacation, even if you are visiting a beachfront luxury hotel.** Here are some calorie-burning tips:
  1. Take walks around the city, theme park, beaches, etc., every day, multiple times a day if you can.
  2. Bring a jump rope, exercise bands, and, of course, your sneakers so you can get in some cardio.
  3. Use the hotel pool. Treading water, swimming laps, and running in place can burn some extra calories while you are enjoying the warm weather and sunshine.
  4. If your hotel has an exercise room, try doing 30 minutes of exercise in the morning to start your day.
  5. Do squats, crunches, pushups, wall sits, and other exercises in your hotel room when you have some spare time.
  6. Walk around the airport with or without your luggage during layovers.

Next time you are on vacation, use these tips to plan ahead for healthy meals, snacks, and exercise. Instead of simply surrendering to vacation weight gain, a good goal is to maintain your weight while you are traveling.

Handling the Holidays

The holidays are a tough time of year, especially when it comes to maintaining your blood sugar. There are parties at work, parties at school, parties with friends, and, oh yes, parties with the family. One thing you know for sure is that there definitely won't be a shortage of food and drinks for any of these festive events, but don't let that be your excuse to splurge!

Waiting for New Year's resolution time to roll around is not an option; research from the NIH (National Institutes of Health) has found that you never lose the few pounds you gain during the holiday season. Take the challenge to fight against the winter (and year-round) weight gain.

Here are some tips to help you conquer the urge to splurge:

- **What you can control:**
    1. Have a high-fiber snack and some water prior to the event so you aren't starving!
    2. Bring a healthy dish to the party.
    3. Make only one trip to the buffet.
    4. Choose the smaller size plate if available.
    5. Load up your plate with high-fiber foods, such as raw vegetables and salad.
    6. Focus on being social at parties. Enjoy the company of family and friends while strategically positioning yourself out of reach of the tempting appetizers.
    7. Drink a full glass of water between any alcoholic drinks. Drinking in moderation is key, 1–2 drinks for women and 2–3 drinks for men. Drinking too much may also lead to eating too much.
    8. Incorporate exercise, especially on the days prior to, the day of, and the days after each event.
- **What you can't control:**
    1. Usually the buffet spread is out of your control. When choosing food from the buffet tables keep an eye out for the colorful foods and beware of the white, creamy foods.
    2. Choose small portions. Try a small spoonful of the other higher-calorie foods only if they are your favorites. Be sure to savor your food!
    3. Choose your sweets wisely; each dessert can have 200–1,200 calories!
    4. Be careful with the appetizers. These little bites of bliss can easily add up in a matter of minutes.
    5. Have your "excuses" ready. One of the best lines is that you are just plain full and maybe you will try some in a little while!
    6. Try to avoid taking home extras, especially the tempting (high-calorie) foods.

Sour-cream dips, cheese balls, little sausages and meatballs, sweets, chocolaty desserts, and alcohol will all be present at the holiday affairs, and so will you! Have your game plan ready.

Late-Night Cravings

If you watch TV at night, you probably have fallen victim to the late-night commercial ads. They may not have sent you to the nearest fast-food joint, but they may have ignited the late-night munchies. You probably were not even hungry, but the seed was planted and got you thinking about food. This is often the cause of late-night eating: Either you were bored or influenced. Either way, you end up eating at a time when your body would prefer not to. Avoid going to bed on a full stomach; when you are sleeping is not necessarily the time to burn those recently ingested calories. Your best bet is to try setting a cut-off time, a time when the kitchen is officially closed, usually 8 P.M. or so.

If you are feeling a craving for a certain food during the day, you may consider trying to find a healthier alternative, such as one of the following:

- Chocolate lovers, get your fix with a batch of homemade popcorn sprinkled with cocoa; fat-free, sugar-free chocolate pudding topped with high-fiber cereal; fat-free frozen yogurt; unflavored almond or coconut milk with a teaspoon of cocoa; or 3–4 dark chocolate–covered almonds.
- Need to cool off? Try something cold and refreshing such as a fruit and spinach salad; sliced fresh cucumbers with a squeeze of lemon; a big bowl of watermelon, cantaloupe, and strawberries; a fresh tomato salad; iced coffee; frozen grapes; nonfat yogurt; frozen yogurt; a fruit smoothie; or cucumber-and-mint-infused water.
- If you are craving salt, grab a small handful of nuts; a bite of a pickle; cauliflower dipped in salsa or pico de gallo; vegetables with hummus or black bean dip; homemade popcorn; vegetables with nonfat cottage cheese or Greek yogurt dips; oven-roasted vegetables; light or nonfat cream cheese with celery; avocado; olives; string cheese; homemade baked sweet potato fries; or 15 almonds. Be sure to read the labels for the actual sodium content, keeping in mind the lower, the better.
- If you are in need of a crunch, grab a bag of baby carrots; celery; cucumbers; green or red peppers; an apple; Kashi Heart to Heart cereal; baked kale chips; or homemade popcorn.
- For that sweet tooth, try grapes; oranges; strawberries; an almond butter banana split; nonfat frozen yogurt; cantaloupe; cherries; peaches; pineapple;

3–4 dark chocolate–covered almonds; a fruit smoothie; a spoonful of almond butter; or homemade popcorn with a drizzle of honey.

When trying to ward off cravings, these healthier options may help. But if you find that you are falling into an unhealthy pattern of cravings that can't be satisfied with a healthier alternative, then it may be best to wean yourself off or stop cold turkey to retrain your taste buds to enjoy the natural flavors of food. If your craving is out of the blue, you may just decide to use this opportunity to splurge, have a small portion of exactly what you want, and then move on with your usual healthy diet. This is the basis of the 80/20 rule. If you are eating healthy at least 80 percent of the time, then you are on track. If you strive for 100 percent of the time, then you are setting yourself up for failure. Keep it real and you can stay on track.

If you choose to drink alcohol, do so in moderation. It is recommended that females limit intake to one drink per day and men limit intake to two drinks per day. It is highly recommended that you have *at least* two alcohol-free days per week. Remember, alcohol provides excessive calories (7 calories per gram) that can increase your blood pressure and contribute to weight gain.

Let's put these calories into perspective:

- 6 ounces wine = 125 calories
- 1 bottle of wine = 530 calories
- 12 ounces light beer = 110 calories
- 6-pack of light beer = 660 calories
- 6 ounces margarita = 320 calories
- 1-ounce shot rum = 65 calories
- 6 mixed drinks with rum and calorie-free mixer = 390 calories

FACT

Alcohol provides empty calories that can lead to weight gain. In addition, it stimulates your appetite, which may lead to overeating and splurging, taking the weight gain another step further. Alcohol also affects blood sugar, especially beer, sweet wine, and mixers that contain carbs. Proceed with caution and in moderation.

Small Substitutions Bring Big Rewards

Healthy substitutions can be a great way to make over a recipe to reduce the fat, sugar, and calories, but it's important to remember that some of the foods still may not be everyday foods. For example, by substituting flaxseed and coconut flour for the flour in your chocolate chip cookies, you are making them a bit healthier; however, they are still chocolate chip cookies and considered a special treat.

Here are some examples of weight-reducing substitutions with added health bonuses:

- ¼ cup egg substitute for 1 egg = 4 pounds per year
  - Bonus: reduction of 5 grams fat and 1.5 grams saturated fat
- 1 orange for 1 cup orange juice = 5 pounds per year
  - Bonus: 5 grams fiber
- Calorie-free spray butter for 1 tablespoon butter = 7 pounds per year
  - Bonus: reduction of 11 grams fat and 7 grams saturated fat
- 1 cup black beans for 3 ounces lean ground beef = 0 pounds per year
  - Bonus: reduction of 14 grams fat and 6 grams saturated fat, not to mention the addition of 15 grams sugar-regulating fiber
- 1 tablespoon avocado for 1 tablespoon mayonnaise = 8 pounds per year
  - Bonus: maximizes your essential fatty acids
- Light ranch dressing for regular ranch dressing = 8 pounds per year
  - Bonus: serve dressing on the side and dip each bite so you consume less
- Cooking spray for 1 tablespoon oil = 12½ pounds per year
  - Bonus: reduction in fat
- ½ cucumber for 1 pita = 15 pounds per year
  - Bonus: nice fresh crunch to serve with hummus
- 1 light English muffin for 1 bagel = 23 pounds per year
  - Bonus: higher in fiber and lower in carbohydrates; will keep blood sugars more stable

These are great examples of everyday ways to make healthier choices. The list can go on and on, but the moral of the story is to choose your foods wisely, looking for foods high in fiber and low in saturated fat and added sugar.

Here are more substitution ideas to incorporate more fruits and healthier fats in your cooking:

❑ Egg replacer: Substitute 1 tablespoon ground flaxseed + 3 tablespoons water. Mix together and allow to sit for 5 minutes, then use in recipe in place of one egg. This exchange eliminates the cholesterol and saturated fat from the egg while substituting a healthier fat profile.
❑ Sour cream: Substitute nonfat, plain Greek yogurt. You will never know the difference, but your body will enjoy the lower fat and calorie switch.
❑ Sugar: Substitute an equal amount of unsweetened applesauce or ⅔ the amount of puréed dates for a naturally sweet alternative.
❑ Oil: Substitute half of the oil with unsweetened applesauce or mashed bananas. This will cut the fat content in half while providing the health benefits of added fruit.
❑ Butter: Substitute avocado when you would normally use butter. Avocado is lower in saturated fat than butter.
❑ White flour: Substitute a portion of the white flour with coconut flour. This will reduce the carbohydrate load of your baked goods.

CHAPTER 5

FAQs and Steps to Success

Anytime you commit to making a lifestyle change, there are going to be roadblocks and struggles, but just remember that the goal is to persevere and set yourself up for success. Questions like "Should I do this?" and "Is this food okay to eat?" will arise. It might be a struggle at times, but continue to work through each situation as it comes up, keeping in mind that in the media and with ongoing research things are always changing. The fundamentals of this diet are stable and hopefully your blood sugar will be as well.

How Can You Increase Your Metabolism?

It is important to realize that there are a handful of things affecting your metabolism that are out of your control, including:

- Your age. Your age keeps going up, but your energy needs are going down. This is a result of hormonal changes as well as a change in muscle and body fat composition.
- Your genetic makeup. Your family's medical history is your medical history, and there is not much you can do about this.
- Your gender. Males tend to have more muscle mass than females; therefore, they are lucky enough to burn more energy.

There are some metabolism-boosting strategies that are in your control, including:

- Your diet. Do your best to avoid dieting; severe calorie restrictions actually slow down the metabolism. This causes the body to transition into a "starvation" state, utilizing fuel very efficiently, no longer burning energy freely.
- Daily exercise. Increasing exercise has a direct effect on your metabolism. Participating in exercise, both aerobic (walking, jogging, biking, swimming, etc.) and anaerobic (lifting weights, sprinting), benefits your metabolism by increasing your muscle mass, which in turn burns more energy.
- Frequent mealtimes. It is important to eat small meals throughout the day to continually nourish your body. Skipping meals slows down the metabolism. Always eat breakfast to jump-start your metabolism for the day, especially because your body went 8–10 hours overnight without food. Remember, your metabolism slows as the day goes on; therefore, dinner should be a light meal and you should try to limit late-night snacking.
- You must drink water. It is an essential component for optimizing your metabolism.
- Get some sleep. Do your best to get to bed at a decent time. The goal is 8–10 hours of sleep every night. Going without sleep puts stress on your

body, increasing your blood sugar. If you are tired, you may not have the energy to prepare your foods or hit the gym.

- Reduce your stress. Prolonged stress reduces your metabolic rate. Try to find ways to reduce the stress in your life, such as meditating; reading a book; going for a walk; listening to calm, relaxing music; taking a warm bath; talking with a friend; dancing; etc.

FACT

Your body requires energy to function. Here is a breakdown of how energy is used in the body. The basal metabolic rate (basically all the things keeping you alive such as breathing and the beating of your heart) uses 60 percent, physical and daily activity use 30 percent, and digestion and absorption of foods use 10 percent, resulting in 100 percent of your total energy expenditure.

What about Adding in Blood Sugar Regulators?

There is quite a bit of research out there about a few specific foods that can be beneficial in reducing your blood sugar, increasing the body's reception of insulin, and therefore reducing your risk of prediabetes. Here are a few favorites to include in your daily routine:

- Cocoa is rich in antioxidants and phytochemicals that can help control insulin. Daily cocoa consumption will also improve your bad cholesterol (LDL) and lower your blood pressure. Since there is such a bond between diabetes and heart disease, this is a win-win!
- Cinnamon has been found to lower blood sugar. It is thought to help the muscle and liver cells respond better to insulin. Although it is certainly not the cure for diabetes, any little bit helps, not to mention the delicious flavor. Shoot for ½ teaspoon per day and let your numbers speak for themselves.
- Blueberries increase your body's sensitivity to insulin. Blueberries have been found to lower blood glucose levels, resulting in better glucose regulation.

- Chia seeds, shelled hemp seeds, and flaxseed provide your body with a high fiber content that helps stabilize changes in your blood sugar. They also improve your response to insulin.
- Vinegar has been reported to help blood sugars remain stable when consumed prior to a meal. Also, vinegar reduces the amount of insulin secreted during a mealtime.

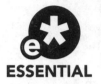

ESSENTIAL

Keeping your blood sugar in the desired range is not so much the magic of one specific food over another but the composition of the food. A diet rich in fiber should lead you to good blood sugar control, as it helps keep your blood sugar from spiking when it is included in your mealtime. Simple enough!

What about Artificial Sweeteners and Sugar Alcohols?

Of course completely avoiding added sugars is best, but are there any other alternatives? There are the artificial sweeteners. Splenda, Sweet'N Low, Equal, and stevia (a nonchemical sweetener) are a few of the most common. All of these sweeteners have been recognized by the Food and Drug Administration as being safe in moderation. The theory is that the body does not digest the artificial sweeteners; therefore, they do not affect your blood sugar control. The latter point is controversial and it seems the jury is still out. Some studies have actually found that artificial sweeteners increase blood sugars, while other studies suggest no change in blood sugars.

If you want to add some sweetness to your meal, your best bet is honey because it's natural. It will increase your blood sugar, but hopefully you are pairing the sweetness with some foods containing healthy fats to slow down the changes in blood sugar with digestion.

FACT

Honey is a super-powered food both inside and out. It has a laundry list of uses, including use as a natural sweetener with antioxidant properties, but it also has been found to help with wound healing, dandruff, and alcohol metabolism, and it may also help improve allergy symptoms and the common cold.

Choosing the Right Sweetener

By now you can see how different sugars affect your blood sugar, and that it is extremely important to limit your added sugar. In a perfect world, your sugar intake would come from only fruits and complex carbohydrates (not artificial or raw sugar). If you wanted to add a little sweetness to your meal, you would reach for some fruit (a.k.a. the preferred sweetener) or possibly honey. But sometimes your lifestyle and food choices make it hard to avoid added sugar or keep it within a healthy range. So then what?

With all the different options out there, you may be wondering how to choose the right sweetener for you. Ask yourself these three questions:

(Note: The following recommendations and statements are based on how different sugars affect both blood sugar and different conditions/ diseases.)

1. Can your body process sugar? One of the best ways to know if your body can process sugar is to ask your doctor to check your hemoglobin A1c.
   - Diabetic: If it is in the diabetic range (more than 6.5), you should pay close attention to all of your carbohydrates; they are necessary to help control your blood sugars. Your best choice is eating high-fiber foods (whole grains, fruits, and vegetables). Avoid all added sugar, and if necessary use artificial sweeteners to control blood sugar levels.
   - Prediabetic: If your hemoglobin A1c is in the prediabetic range (5.6–6.4), or you have a family history of diabetes, blood sugar management is essential to change your direction in order to prevent diabetes. Your best choices are also high-fiber carbohydrates and limiting added sugars, with use of artificial sweeteners if needed to maintain blood sugar levels.

- Healthy blood sugar: If your hemoglobin A1c is normal (less than 5.5), meaning your body is processing sugar well, then your best sweetener choices are high-fiber carbohydrates and limiting your intake of added sugar in accordance with the American Heart Association's recommendations. High-fiber carbohydrate choices such as fruits and whole grains are acceptable, as well as limiting added sugar for a healthy lifestyle.

2. Are you pregnant?
   - Gestational diabetes is a concern during pregnancy. Your best sweetener choice is similar to that of a diabetic or prediabetic: eating high-fiber foods, including whole grains and fruits (limit fruit to 1 small serving at a time), as well as occasional use of artificial sweeteners, with the exception of saccharin, as it crosses the placenta barrier to your baby.

3. Do you have underlying health conditions?
   - If you are overweight, you are at a higher risk for diabetes and heart disease. It is essential to lose weight. High-fiber food choices will help satisfy your appetite sooner, lowering your total calorie intake for the day and resulting in weight loss. Occasional use of artificial sweeteners may also be beneficial to help reduce overall calorie intake to help with weight loss.
   - If you have high triglycerides or low HDL cholesterol, you are at increased risk for heart disease and stroke. Your best option is to drastically reduce your added sugar intake to lower your triglycerides, replacing these foods with high-fiber foods that may help with lowering your LDL and VLDL cholesterol and keeping your heart healthy.

What about the Glycemic Index?

The glycemic index is a measure of how different carbohydrates affect your blood sugar. Researchers have assigned a glycemic index value to foods to represent the how fast or slow the blood sugar changes with intake of each food. The process of assigning glycemic index values to foods is done by comparing intakes of the specified food to sugar and observing the effects on the person's blood sugars. Foods that break down rapidly have high glycemic index values, and foods that break down slowly have lower glycemic index values.

There are several factors that affect a food's glycemic index value. The composition of the food determines how fast or slow the blood sugar is going to respond. High-fiber foods, including fruits, vegetables, beans, and whole grains with fibrous pieces, take longer to digest, similar to the slower digestion of fat, resulting in better blood sugar control. At the opposite end of the spectrum is food with small particles that are broken down quickly, such as finely milled flour; these foods have a high glycemic index value (a.k.a. sugar spike).

For the purposes of the blood sugar diet, it is nice to know about the glycemic index, but it should not be your focus. The goal is to combine foods in a way that balances fiber, carbs, and fat in order to control your blood sugar. You definitely do not need another thing to worry about.

Do You Have to Avoid Meat, Dairy, and Gluten?

The simple answer is no, you do not need to eliminate meat, dairy, and gluten. All foods can fit into your healthier lifestyle, but these should be the exceptions rather than the staples in your diet. You should have these three foods in small portions. Meat and dairy foods are known to have high saturated fat content, while plant-based proteins do not, and are therefore a much better option for you and your heart.

Gluten is the protein found in wheat, rye, and barley, and sometimes it cross-contaminates into oats during processing. A gluten-free diet is appropriate for someone with the medical condition celiac disease, but it is not a requirement for most, especially those with prediabetes or type 2 diabetes. There are personal testimonials out there supporting improvements in health with the gluten-free diet, but at this point the research is just not there to support it. When it comes to gluten, it is not that it is restricted on this diet, but you should be aware that most of the foods containing gluten (pastas, breads, cereals) are usually rich in carbs and should be limited. These types of carbs can quickly add up to an excess and lead to weight gain. Remember, focus on getting your carbs from the better, not-so-obvious sources: beans, vegetables, and fruits.

FACT

Type 1 diabetes and celiac disease are both autoimmune diseases that often present in tandem. But type 2 diabetes does not have the same connection. Therefore, a gluten-free diet may be appropriate for type 1 diabetics but not type 2.

Essentials of Exercise

Exercise can help your body (and mind) become healthier for so many reasons, but there are a few benefits that directly help you reduce your risk of diabetes. One benefit is weight management. Daily exercise will help you slowly start burning fat, building muscle, and burning more calories to achieve a healthier body weight. The second benefit is the improvement in blood sugar control. When you exercise, your body uses the glucose (sugar) in your blood for energy, thereby lowering your blood sugar. This process also improves the body's response to insulin, becoming more responsive not only during but also after your workout, which all translates into better sugar metabolism.

The number-one excuse for skipping a workout is that you just don't have enough time. Usually this line is followed by more excuses including school schedules, work schedules, household chores, or lack of sleep. Time is valuable. In order to utilize every opportunity you have for a little calorie burn, you need to be creative.

Here are some tips for finding ways to burn some extra calories:

- Use your kids and their energy level to your advantage!
    1. Include an afterschool activity that involves a walk, run, bike ride, race, or a mean game of tag.
    2. If you have a small child or baby, take a walk with him in your arms. The extra weight adds to the amount of calories you burn!
    3. Play follow the leader, and when it's your turn, try including funny plyometrics (e.g., high knees, power skipping, jump squats). Your kids will love your ideas!

4. Take your kids swimming. There are a lot of calories to burn at the pool using the water's resistance, including some simple moves such as treading water, leg kicks, running, and jumping.

- Work out at work.
  1. Take a stair break. Find a route to the bathroom that includes a few flights of stairs.
  2. Flex your muscles and your mind. Try sitting up straight in your chair and flexing your abs, then lift your feet off the floor in repetitions. With your knees glued together, try swinging your feet to each side (you should feel this move around your upper thighs and waist!).
  3. When possible, stand up. You burn more calories standing than sitting!
  4. Try a lunch workout. While your lunch is cooking in the microwave, use this time to do squats and lunges. These moves work your large muscle groups, and therefore burn more calories.

- Do some calorie-burning household moves.
  1. Grocery groove. Unload groceries to music. While you are putting things away, try lifting different foods (e.g., canned items, watermelons, and cantaloupe) in repetition. Some easy lifts to begin with include bicep curls, side raises, side twists, and above-the-head raises.
  2. Power vacuum. Incorporate lunges as you vacuum each area of your house.
  3. Two minutes of laundry fun. For each load of your never-ending laundry, try incorporating two minutes of strength moves, such as wall sits, lunges, stairs, squats, and explosive jumps.
  4. Bathroom breaks. When cleaning the bathroom, scrub the tub clean with different arm moves and reps of pushups.

- Hit the gym.
  1. Make the most of your workout by doing interval training. For example, do a few minutes of running, stairs, or elliptical, and then a few reps of weights.
  2. Join a class. Cardio and cycling classes are a great way to keep yourself accountable.
  3. If you don't have gym access, try shadowboxing in front of the mirror, dancing, or going out for a jog.

- Burn calories at bedtime.
  1. Work your abs in bed. Try doing v-ups, ab crunches, and the bicycle in reps of 20 each every night.
  2. Tooth-brushing wall sits is just what it sounds like. Dentists recommend brushing for two minutes every morning and night.
  3. Prayer time plank. When taking time to meditate over your day, don't be afraid to do so in plank position. Drop down onto your elbows/forearms with a flat, flexed body, up on your toes. Even 30 seconds will allow you to feel the burn.
  4. Shower squats. Just be sure you have your footing.
  5. Bedside dips. Sitting on the edge of your bed, put your hands down next to you with your arms at a 90-degree angle. Slowly lift your bottom off the side of the bed, and using your triceps dip down and back up in repetition.

These are just a few occasions to sneak in some calorie-burning moves. You can always bust out some dance moves or flexing in the car, in the shower, or during commercial breaks. Challenge yourself to go out of your way to burn more calories. You will soon find that you do have the time!

Venturing Out of Your Comfort Zone

If you have a hard time even conceiving the idea that you need to make a change, you should take this challenge step by step. Do not try to make a 180-degree change overnight. Doing that, like trying most fad diets, will end in an ultimate fail. Make changes you are comfortable with and eventually you will convert yourself over to a healthier lifestyle. The key is to gain some momentum. If weight loss is your goal, then start with increasing your intake of fruits and vegetables. If you are successful in increasing your intake to 7–11 servings per day, this will offset your usual intake and get the weight loss ball rolling.

Try working your way out of your comfort zone by taking the challenge of trying a few new foods:

- Chia seeds, flaxseed, and shelled hemp seeds—These seeds are lower-carbohydrate grains, packed with protein, fiber, and essential fats. Researchers have found that adding flaxseed to your diet is linked to lowering your blood cholesterol as much as a cholesterol medication. With heart disease topping the list of causes of death, it seems that adding a little ground flaxseed to your meal may be a good idea.

- Green chilies, curry, garlic, rosemary, basil, cilantro, olives, capers, and sun-dried tomatoes are all lower-calorie, flavor-boosting foods, bound to make your high-fiber dinner taste perfect.

- Cinnamon—You can improve your glucose metabolism if you consume just ¼–1 teaspoon of cinnamon a day. This means that it helps your body use insulin efficiently, moving the glucose out of your blood and into cells for energy. Eating cinnamon on a daily basis will help keep your blood sugar level stable, and will reduce your risk of diabetes.

- Sweet potatoes—When compared to the ordinary white potato, the sweet potato is lower in carbohydrates and calories, and provides a powerful punch of antioxidants that are associated with disease prevention. The lower carbohydrate content and the bonus fiber content keep your blood sugar stable, and you'll be satisfying your appetite with fewer calories, while helping to keep your body at a healthy weight and your metabolism functioning at its best.

- Hummus, walnuts, almonds, and avocado—These foods provide mostly good fats (essential, polyunsaturated, and monounsaturated) that have been found to lower bad cholesterol and increase good cholesterol. This is important for everyone, but especially those with diabetes or those who are overweight and at risk for heart disease.

- Cocoa, dates, and honey provide natural sweetness without chemical manipulation.

- Dried beans and lentils—Venture out of the canned bean zone! Simply soak those beans overnight, drain the water, refill the water, and cook. Piece of cake!

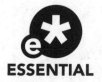

ESSENTIAL

Take a chance on a few new foods. Whether it was Brussels sprouts, beets, or raspberries that you swore off when you were a child, it is now time to grow up and give these superfoods another chance. You may be surprised that your taste buds have grown up, too.

Set Yourself Up for Success

You need to know where you stand in terms of your diet, exercise, and mental health. All three are important components of weight management success, but if one is out of balance, you need to be aware and make the changes to improve the balance. This is just like when you exercise without drinking enough water. The lack of proper hydration may be slowing down your metabolism, leaving all of the sweat and frustration in the gym and your weight unchanged.

You need to know what changes you can make to maximize your metabolism. If you are falling short or in excess of any key nutrients, your metabolism may be slowing down while your weight may be trending up. For example, if you have unique fat needs based on weight and medical history, taking in too much or too little fat may result in weight gain.

You need to find a plan you can stick with over time. This plan needs to include multiple small but powerful changes that can improve your body's metabolism for the long term. You also need to keep yourself accountable. You can do anything for a week or two, but sticking with something over a long period of time (a.k.a. lifestyle change) takes a lot of accountability. Friends who work out or take on a healthy eating initiative together are more successful than a person taking on a new healthy eating or exercise plan alone.

Here are some things to consider when you are formulating your game plan for success:

1. Plan out your week, making a point to identify all of the potential areas of temptation and possibilities of splurging. Then plan how you are going to offset these splurges (e.g., choosing a lighter lunch, doing an extra caloric-burning workout, picking and choosing your splurges carefully, etc.).
2. Prepare quick, healthy meals and snacks to have on hand when you are in a hurry.
3. Make breakfast and/or lunch the night before to help save time.
4. When you are feeling stressed or bored and get the urge to eat, take 10 or 20 minutes to see if you are really hungry before eating. If you are not sure, try crunching on some carrots, cucumbers, or celery.

5. Drink plenty of water to keep hydrated and on the move. Avoid caffein-ated and sugary beverages and drink alcohol in moderation.

6. Keep a positive attitude when it comes to stress. Focus on things you can control, not on things out of your control. At the very least, laugh (a lot)! Laughing burns calories.

7. Fit in fitness. Working out releases endorphins, which help you feel relaxed.

8. Share your feelings of stress with a close friend or family member to help release some tension. They probably have some to relieve as well.

ALERT

It can be extremely difficult and frustrating to make lifestyle changes and stick to them. Try to stay balanced. Take each day as a new opportunity to follow the blood sugar diet and improve your health.

CHAPTER 6

Breakfast of Champions

Baked Apple Cinnamon Oatmeal Muffins

This is a quick and easy batch recipe that can be made on Sunday,
placed in the freezer, and eaten for breakfast throughout the week.

INGREDIENTS | MAKES 12 MUFFINS

1 cup steel cut oats

½ cup ground flaxseed

½ teaspoon baking powder

½ teaspoon salt

1 teaspoon cinnamon

½ cup unsweetened coconut milk

1 large egg

½ medium banana, mashed

1 teaspoon honey

1 medium apple, diced

⅓ cup chopped walnuts

1. Preheat oven to 450°F. Spray muffin tin with cooking spray.

2. In a medium bowl, combine oats, flaxseed, baking powder, salt, and cinnamon. Add coconut milk, egg, banana, and honey, mixing well. Then fold in apple and walnuts.

3. Spoon mixture into muffin tin. Bake 20 minutes.

Brussels for Breakfast

Vegetables are not commonly eaten for breakfast, but by including sweet potatoes and Brussels sprouts in your egg scramble, you are on the right path to achieving your goal of 7–11 servings of fruits and vegetables per day.

INGREDIENTS | SERVES 4

2 medium sweet potatoes, diced

1 medium red onion, peeled and diced

2 cups quartered Brussels sprouts

2 tablespoons olive oil

8 egg whites, whisked

¼ teaspoon salt

¼ teaspoon ground black pepper

1. In a medium skillet, sauté sweet potatoes, onion, and Brussels sprouts in oil over medium heat for 20–25 minutes until potatoes and Brussels sprouts are softened and caramelized.

2. Meanwhile, spray a small skillet with cooking spray and heat pan over medium heat. Once pan is warm, add egg whites and stir with a fork until light and fluffy.

3. Add egg whites to sweet potatoes and Brussels sprouts mixture, lightly seasoning with salt and pepper.

Honey Butter Banana

Even though breakfast is the most important meal of the day, many people commonly skip it due to a lack of time. You can make this quick and easy breakfast on the go, even in the biggest rush. Prep time for this breakfast treat is 4 minutes max!

INGREDIENTS | SERVES 1

1 medium banana

2 teaspoons almond butter

1 teaspoon ground flaxseed and/or shelled hemp seeds

½ teaspoon cinnamon

½ teaspoon honey

1. Slice banana lengthwise ¾ of the way through. Spread almond butter between the two halves and gently press together.

2. Sprinkle flaxseed and/or hemp seeds and cinnamon over banana, then drizzle with honey. Slice into coin-sized bites.

Add Those Seeds

Flaxseed and hemp seeds add both protein and fat to this recipe. Both of these macronutrients help round out the carbohydrate load of the banana, slowing down the digestion and absorption of the sugars and resulting in better blood sugar control.

Buckwheat Pancakes

These pancakes deliver a heartier, more intense flavor than your traditional pancakes.
Try adding sliced bananas or berries to the batter for a sweeter pancake!

INGREDIENTS | SERVES 2

1 cup whole-wheat flour
½ cup buckwheat flour
1½ teaspoons baking powder
2 egg whites
¼ cup apple juice concentrate
1¼–1½ cups skim milk or milk substitute

1. Sift flours and baking powder together in a medium bowl. In another medium bowl, combine egg whites, apple juice concentrate, and 1¼ cups milk. Add milk mixture to dry ingredients; mix well, but do not over-mix. Add remaining milk if necessary to reach desired consistency.

2. Treat a griddle pan with nonstick spray, or use a large nonstick skillet. Heat over medium heat. Ladle the batter onto the hot pan with a ¼-cup measuring scoop, and cook for 2–3 minutes. When bubbles appear on the surface of the pancake, flip and cook for 2 minutes or until browned. Repeat until all pancake batter is used.

Green Egg Breakfast Wrap

This is not quite the breakfast Dr. Seuss was talking about, but the flavor and fiber in this green-tinted breakfast is sure to please the taste buds and keep you feeling satisfied all morning long.

INGREDIENTS | SERVES 1

2 egg whites, whisked

½ medium avocado, mashed

1 teaspoon prepared pesto

1 cup chopped spinach

1 high-fiber tortilla

1. In a medium skillet that has been sprayed with cooking spray, cook egg whites over medium heat approximately 4–5 minutes.

2. Meanwhile, spread avocado and pesto on tortilla. Add egg whites and spinach, then roll up and serve.

Find That Fiber

Choose your tortilla carefully. Look for a fiber-rich tortilla that has 3 grams of fiber or more per tortilla. The increased fiber content helps slow down the digestion of food, which is the key to keeping blood sugars stable and warding off diabetes.

Roasted Coconut Berry Parfait

The natural flavors of coconut, berries, and honey give this parfait sweetness without the sugar spike!

INGREDIENTS | SERVES 1

¼ cup unsweetened coconut flakes

1 cup plain, nonfat Greek yogurt

1 cup fresh or frozen mixed berries
(raspberries, strawberries, blueberries)

2 tablespoons ground flaxseed

½ teaspoon honey

½ teaspoon unsweetened cocoa powder

Freeze and Be Frugal!

Save money by buying mass amounts of berries when they're on sale during the peak season and freezing them. Strawberries are best March through August, and the other berries are best June through August.

1. Preheat oven to 350°F. Spread coconut flakes in a thin layer in a shallow baking dish. Bake for 3–5 minutes until lightly golden. Keep a close eye on the coconut, as it will burn quickly.

2. In a small bowl, prepare parfait by layering ½ of the Greek yogurt, berries, coconut, and flaxseed, and repeat with remaining ½. Top with drizzle of honey and sprinkle of cocoa powder.

Egg-cellent Sandwich

If you are looking to keep your cholesterol low, substitute two egg whites for the whole egg.

INGREDIENTS | SERVES 1

1 large egg or 2 egg whites
1 high-fiber English muffin
¼ cup shredded pepper jack cheese
1 tablespoon sun-dried tomatoes
¼ cup spinach leaves

Egg Yolks in Moderation

The general recommendation is to keep your cholesterol intake under 200 milligrams per day. The good news is that you can eat one egg per day and stay within that guideline. Each egg contains 200 milligrams of cholesterol. You just need to be careful if you are eating additional sources of cholesterol, specifically any animal meat or product.

1. Preheat oven to 350°F.

2. In a small skillet sprayed with cooking spray, crack egg and cook approximately 5 minutes on each side.

3. Toast English muffin in oven for approximately 5–10 minutes or use a toaster oven to toast until golden brown. Remove from oven or toaster and top with cooked egg and shredded cheese. Then top with sun-dried tomatoes and spinach.

Sweet Breakfast Quesadilla

Vary the flavors by trying peanut, cashew, or sunflower seed butter in place of the almond butter. Nut and seed butters are great sources of protein and are rich in healthy fats.

INGREDIENTS | SERVES 1

1 high-fiber tortilla

2 teaspoons almond butter

½ medium banana, sliced

4 strawberries, sliced

¼ cup blueberries

¼ teaspoon honey

1 teaspoon ground flaxseed

⅛ teaspoon unsweetened cocoa (optional)

1. Assemble quesadilla by spreading tortilla with almond butter, topping with fruits, and folding in half.

2. In a medium skillet sprayed with cooking spray, heat quesadilla until almond butter is melted, 2–3 minutes.

3. Drizzle with honey and sprinkle with flaxseed and cocoa if desired.

Omega-3 versus Omega-6

Sometimes the lower the number, the better. That is the case with the omegas! The American diet seems to be extra rich in omega-6 fatty acids, relative to the lower content of the omega-3s. The desired ratio for omega-6 to omega-3 is 4:1 or lower. Eating flaxseed and hemp seeds helps to equalize that balancing act. Try adding these seeds to almost anything.

Crustless Zucchini and Artichoke Quiche

This breakfast delivers the cheesy, delicious flavors of quiche without the carbohydrate- and fat-laden crust. Try serving with chopped tomatoes and basil on the side.

INGREDIENTS | SERVES 4

1 tablespoon olive oil

¼ cup chopped onion

¾ cup grated zucchini

1 cup canned artichoke hearts cut into ½" pieces

1½ cups grated light Cheddar cheese

2 large eggs

2 egg whites

½ cup fat-free cottage cheese

¼ teaspoon cayenne pepper

¼ teaspoon salt

⅛ teaspoon freshly ground black pepper

1. Preheat oven to 375°F. Spray a 9" pie plate with cooking spray. In a large nonstick skillet, heat olive oil over medium heat; add onion and sauté until translucent, 7–10 minutes.

2. Add zucchini and artichoke hearts; cook an additional 3 minutes.

3. Sprinkle grated cheese in bottom of pie plate; add cooked vegetables on top of cheese.

4. In a small bowl, whisk together eggs, egg whites, cottage cheese, cayenne pepper, salt, and black pepper; pour over vegetables.

5. Bake 35–40 minutes or until set and a toothpick inserted in the center comes out clean.

Honey Oat Breakfast Bites

Make a batch of these breakfast bites on Sunday. Place in the freezer in single, portioned baggies. Each night move one serving to the refrigerator so you are ready to go in the morning.

INGREDIENTS | SERVES 6

1¼ cups chopped walnuts, divided
½ cup dates
1½ cups quick-cooking steel cut oats
½ cup ground flaxseed
3 tablespoons honey
1 teaspoon unsweetened cocoa powder
1 teaspoon vanilla extract

1. In a food processor, purée 1 cup walnuts until creamy. Add dates, and pulse a few times to slightly purée dates.

2. Spoon mixture into a bowl, mix in remaining ingredients, including remaining ¼ cup walnuts. Mix all ingredients well.

3. Form into bite-sized balls and refrigerate or freeze.

Avocado Toast

Avocado serves as a rich, "buttery" spread for your morning toast. Top with sautéed spinach and fresh tomatoes and be on your merry way!

INGREDIENTS | SERVES 1

2 cups chopped spinach

1 teaspoon olive oil

⅛ teaspoon sea salt

¼ teaspoon garlic powder

1 slice high-fiber bread

½ small ripe avocado, mashed

½ medium Roma tomato, sliced

1. In a medium saucepan over medium heat, sauté spinach in olive oil, seasoned with salt and garlic powder, for approximately 2–4 minutes until cooked.

2. Meanwhile, toast bread, then spread with avocado and top with sautéed spinach and tomato slices.

Avocado As a Butter Sub

Substituting avocado for butter, cream cheese, sour cream, or mayo in a recipe is an unbelievable tactic to help reduce not only the obvious saturated fat (a.k.a. the bad fat) but also total fat, calories, and sodium.

Lemon Berry Chia Breakfast Pudding

This recipe is best prepared at night and stored in a Mason jar in the refrigerator. While you sleep, the chia seeds will go to work to transform this mixture into a delicious fresh fruit pudding.

INGREDIENTS | SERVES 1

1 cup unsweetened almond milk

3 tablespoons chia seeds

1 teaspoon ground flaxseed

1 teaspoon honey

1 teaspoon lemon juice

1 teaspoon grated lemon zest

½ cup berries

1. Pour almond milk into container with cover. Add chia seeds, stirring well. Mix in flaxseed, honey, lemon juice, and lemon zest. Cover and store in the refrigerator overnight.

2. Top with berries and additional flaxseed if desired.

Cha-Cha-Cha Chia!

When you hear the word *chia*, you probably think of the Chia Pet, but there is a whole new chia on the block, one that serves a much greater purpose for your health! Chia seeds are rich in antioxidants, which fight the bad guys in your body that can lead to cancer. They also help regulate your blood sugar due to the high fiber and low carbohydrate content.

Flax Banana Bread

Using flaxseed in this recipe reduces the amount of flour (carbs) while increasing the fiber and healthy fat to balance out the meal and your blood sugar.

INGREDIENTS | SERVES 12

¾ cup all-purpose flour

½ cup coconut flour

¾ cup ground flaxseed

⅔ cup sugar (or Splenda)

2 teaspoons baking powder

¼ teaspoon salt

1 cup mashed bananas (about 3 medium)

2 large eggs

¼ cup skim milk or milk substitute

¼ cup canola oil

½ teaspoon vanilla extract

⅓ cup chopped walnuts and/or chocolate chips

1. Preheat oven to 350°F. Spray 9" × 5" loaf pan with cooking spray.

2. In a large bowl, mix together flours, flaxseed, sugar, baking powder, and salt. In a medium bowl, combine bananas, eggs, milk, oil, and vanilla, mixing well. Mix dry ingredients into banana mixture until just moistened. Fold in nuts and/or chocolate chips.

3. Pour mixture into prepared loaf pan. Bake 50–55 minutes until brown and a toothpick inserted in center comes out clean. Cool for 20 minutes, then remove from pan.

Mushroom and Kale Quiche

Egg whites give this breakfast a bump in protein, without the added fat or cholesterol of the yolk.

INGREDIENTS | SERVES 4

½ medium white onion, peeled and diced

2 cloves garlic, peeled and minced

1 teaspoon olive oil

8 ounces portabella mushrooms, sliced

2 bunches kale, stemmed and chopped

8 egg whites

¼ teaspoon sea salt

¼ teaspoon ground black pepper

½ cup shredded Swiss cheese

1 medium green onion, sliced (optional)

1. In a medium skillet over medium heat, sauté onion and garlic in olive oil 3–4 minutes, then add mushrooms. Continue to sauté mixture an additional 8–10 minutes until mushrooms have become smaller and lightly browned.

2. Meanwhile, preheat oven to 350°F. Spray casserole dish with cooking spray. Fill dish with kale and mushroom mixture.

3. In a medium bowl, whisk egg whites with salt and pepper. Stir in cheese and pour over vegetables.

4. Cook 40–50 minutes until lightly browned and the center of casserole is solid when poked with a fork.

5. Top with additional shredded cheese and sliced green onion if desired.

Breakfast Salad

This salad is virtually a smoothie before it hits the blender. Enjoy fresh vegetables and fruits, balanced with Greek yogurt (good source of protein) and walnuts and almond butter (good sources of fat).

INGREDIENTS | SERVES 1

2 cups chopped spinach

½ medium banana

4 strawberries, diced

1 medium kiwi, peeled and diced

1 medium mango, peeled and diced

½ cup plain, nonfat Greek yogurt

1 tablespoon almond butter

½ teaspoon honey

1 teaspoon chopped walnuts

1. In a medium bowl, combine spinach, banana, strawberries, kiwi, and mango.

2. Combine yogurt, almond butter, and honey in food processor, blending until smooth. Drizzle over salad, then top with walnuts.

Color Your Plate

In order to get your daily 7–11 servings of fruits and vegetables in your diet, use color as your meal-making guide. Try to include several different colors when making your meals, just like this recipe, which includes a combination of red, yellow, and green. The more colors you add, the more vitamins, minerals, antioxidants, and phytochemicals your meals will provide.

Quinoa Berry Breakfast

Quinoa is high in protein and essential amino acids, making it an excellent choice to fuel your body in the morning. This quinoa porridge is a great alternative to traditional oatmeal.

INGREDIENTS | SERVES 4

1 cup quinoa
2 cups water
¼ cup chopped walnuts
1 teaspoon cinnamon
2 cups berries
¼ cup unsweetened almond milk
(optional)

1. Rinse quinoa in fine-mesh sieve before cooking. Place quinoa, water, walnuts, and cinnamon in a 1½-quart saucepan; bring to a boil. Reduce heat to low; cover and cook 15 minutes or until all water has been absorbed.

2. Add berries and top each serving with 1 tablespoon almond milk if desired.

Single Serving Quick Tip

Use this basic recipe to make four servings at once. Refrigerate any leftover portions; microwave 1–1½ minutes on high for single portions as needed. Use cooked quinoa within 3 days. Try other berries, nuts, or spices such as ginger or nutmeg to vary this nutritious breakfast cereal.

Triple B–Breakfast Bean Bowl

Get your weekend off to a great start with a fiber-loaded breakfast scramble.

INGREDIENTS | SERVES 4

½ medium white onion, peeled and diced

1 tablespoon olive oil

2 medium sweet potatoes, peeled and diced

8 egg whites, whisked

2 cups prepared refried beans

1 medium avocado

1 medium Roma tomato, diced

Green salsa (optional)

2 roasted green chilies, diced (optional)

1. In a medium skillet, sauté onion in olive oil over medium heat, approximately 8–10 minutes. Add potatoes and continue cooking until soft, another 15 minutes.

2. Meanwhile, in a medium skillet sprayed with cooking spray, cook egg whites over medium heat, approximately 4–5 minutes.

3. Heat beans in a small saucepan over medium heat, stirring often.

4. Serve in 4 serving bowls, layered with potatoes, beans, eggs, avocado, and tomatoes. Add green salsa and chilies if desired.

Oatmeal Deluxe

Add extra coconut milk to this recipe to turn it into a drinkable meal for a breakfast on the go.

INGREDIENTS | SERVES 4

¼ cup wheat germ
½ cup walnuts
1 cup quick-cooking steel cut oats
¼ cup ground flaxseed
1 tablespoon cinnamon
2 tablespoons honey
1 cup unsweetened coconut milk

What's All the Hype about Steel Cut Oatmeal?

All brands of oatmeal come from the same whole-grain source: oats. The major difference between instant, rolled, and steel cut oats is how much they are processed. The more they are processed, the easier the body can digest and absorb the carbohydrates, resulting in increased blood sugar. That is why the least processed version, steel cut, is the most satisfying for both hunger and blood sugar balance.

1. Preheat oven to 350°F. Spread wheat germ and walnuts in a thin layer in a shallow baking dish. Bake 5–10 minutes until lightly golden. Keep a close eye, as the wheat germ will burn quickly.

2. Meanwhile, prepare oats with water according to package instructions. Once oatmeal is ready, mix in flaxseed, cinnamon, and honey.

3. Divide oatmeal into 4 serving dishes. Top each serving with toasted wheat germ and walnuts. Add a splash of coconut milk to each.

Veggie Lover Omelet

Reduce this recipe depending on how many omelets you want to make. Remember, the more veggies you can squeeze into this omelet, the better!

INGREDIENTS | SERVES 4

1 medium onion, peeled and diced

1 medium red pepper, seeded and diced

2 tablespoons olive oil

1 cup mushrooms

½ medium zucchini, diced

2 medium Roma tomatoes, diced

8 egg whites, whisked

½ cup shredded Cheddar cheese

1. In a medium skillet, sauté onion and red pepper in olive oil over medium heat. Cook 5 minutes, then add mushrooms and zucchini. After 10 minutes, add tomatoes, cover, and remove from heat.

2. Meanwhile, spray a medium skillet with cooking spray. Heat pan over medium heat, pour ¼ of egg whites into pan and cook 3–4 minutes. Add ¼ of vegetable mixture and 2 tablespoons cheese, then fold egg in half and continue to cook another 2–4 minutes.

3. Repeat step 2 to make 4 omelets.

Whole-Wheat Blueberry Muffins

Because these muffins have very little fat, they'll want to stick to the paper liners or the muffin tin. Your best bet is to skip the muffin liners and be sure to spray the muffin tin well. Letting them cool before removing them will help with easy removal.

INGREDIENTS | MAKES APPROXIMATELY 18 MUFFINS

2 cups whole-wheat flour

1 cup all-purpose flour

1¼ cups sugar

1 tablespoon baking powder

1 teaspoon salt

1½ cups milk or milk substitute

½ cup applesauce

½ teaspoon vanilla extract

2 cups blueberries

Making Vegan Muffins

Got a favorite muffin recipe? Try making it vegan! Use a commercial brand vegan egg replacer in place of the eggs, and substitute a vegan soy margarine and almond milk for the butter and regular milk. Voilà!

1. Preheat oven to 400°F.

2. In a large bowl, combine flours, sugar, baking powder, and salt. Set aside.

3. In a separate small bowl, whisk together milk, applesauce, and vanilla until well mixed.

4. Add the wet ingredients to the dry ingredients, stirring just until mixed. Gently fold in half of the blueberries.

5. Spoon batter into greased muffin tins, filling each tin about ⅔ full. Sprinkle remaining blueberries on top of muffins.

6. Bake for 20–25 minutes or until lightly golden brown on top.

CHAPTER 7

Superfood Smoothies

Super Strawberry Smoothie

You can use fresh or frozen strawberries and bananas in this recipe.

INGREDIENTS | SERVES 1

¼ cup unsweetened coconut milk

½ cup unsweetened applesauce

4 strawberries, stems removed

1 medium banana

1 tablespoon ground flaxseed

1 tablespoon wheat germ

Add all ingredients to the blender and blend until smooth.

The Secret to a Super Smooth Smoothie

When preparing your smoothie, it is best to add the liquid first. This allows the food processor blades free reign to purée your superfood concoction to perfection.

Chia-C Water

This is not just your average glass of water; it is super-powered with super soluble fiber (the good one that lowers your cholesterol) and is loaded with vitamin C, which will help fend off any illness coming your way.

INGREDIENTS | SERVES 1

2 cups water

Juice of 1 medium lemon

1 tablespoon chia seeds

1 medium tangerine, peeled, sectioned, and cut in half

Mix together all ingredients in the blender. Cover, shake well, and refrigerate 12–24 hours to allow chia seeds to soften.

Fruit Infusion

Being that most people are chronically dehydrated, increasing your water intake is an essential step in improving your metabolism. Infuse your water with fruits, vegetables, and herbs. Simply add watermelon, cantaloupe, lemons, limes, berries, cucumber, mint, or whatever else you have in your refrigerator to a pitcher of water and enjoy.

Wake Up Coffee Lovers Smoothie

Get your day started right with this combination of coffee, cocoa, almond, and cinnamon. You may try brewing the coffee the night before and refrigerating in preparation for this quick wake-up smoothie!

INGREDIENTS | SERVES 2

1 cup brewed coffee, chilled

2 cups ice

½ cup unsweetened coconut milk

2 tablespoons ground flaxseed

2 tablespoons wheat germ

2 teaspoons honey

1 tablespoon almond butter

1 teaspoon unsweetened cocoa powder

1 teaspoon cinnamon

Add all ingredients to the blender and blend until smooth.

Mango Smoothie

Mango and banana make this smoothie so smooth and naturally sweet.

INGREDIENTS | SERVES 1

2 tablespoons water

1 medium mango, peeled, sliced, and core removed

1 medium banana, frozen

1 tablespoon ground flaxseed

Add all ingredients to the blender and blend until smooth.

Mango Madness

If you haven't branched out into the world of mangos, you have got to give them a try. It seems the most intimidating part about mangos is cutting them up. Here is a quick tutorial: Using a serrated knife, gently slice just under the skin to remove it. Once the skin is removed, start slicing the mango, removing as much of the meat of the mango as possible, leaving the long, flat core behind. For this smoothie, you can just throw it in as is, but for other recipes you may want to dice into smaller pieces.

Raspberry Tart Morning Start

Raspberries and lime join to make a sweet and tart smoothie that will please all of your taste buds!

INGREDIENTS | SERVES 3

1 cup plain, nonfat Greek yogurt
1 cup chopped romaine lettuce
2 pints raspberries
½ medium lime, peeled

Fight Cancer with Sweetness

Limes and raspberries are extremely powerful additions to any diet. Rich in antioxidants and nutrients, these two fruits pair up to keep your immune system running at its best.

1. Pour ½ cup yogurt into a blender, followed by the romaine, raspberries, and lime. Blend.

2. Continue adding remaining yogurt while blending until desired texture is achieved.

Nutty for Oatmeal Smoothie

If you don't have cooked oatmeal ready, try taking uncooked oats and processing them in a food processor before preparing this smoothie.

INGREDIENTS | SERVES 1

½ cup unsweetened coconut milk
1 medium banana
½ cup cooked oatmeal
¼ cup walnuts
1 teaspoon cinnamon
1 teaspoon honey
1 tablespoon ground flaxseed

Add all ingredients to the blender and blend until smooth.

Freeze Those Nuts!

Nuts are great sources of healthy fats, but unfortunately those fats go bad after too much time stored at room temperature. You can extend the life of most nuts by storing them in the freezer 1–2 years past their sell-by date!

Berry Good Smoothie

This smoothie is the perfect balance of high-fiber fruits, protein-rich Greek yogurt, and healthy-fat-rich flaxseed. This smoothie will surely get your day started right!

INGREDIENTS | SERVES 1

1 cup frozen berries
1 cup plain, nonfat Greek yogurt
½ cup applesauce
1 tablespoon ground flaxseed
1 medium banana

Add all ingredients to the blender and blend until smooth.

"Why Greek?" You Ask

Greek yogurt is special in that on average it contains double the protein and half the carbs compared to regular yogurt. Not enough to convince you to try it? Research has also found a link between yogurt consumption and weight loss. Try getting one nonfat serving daily and see what happens!

Very Veggie Smoothie

Spinach acts as the green base of this smoothie. But you'll find plentiful colors—and tastes—coming from the addition of carrots, celery, tomato, green onion, and parsley.

INGREDIENTS | SERVES 3

1 cup chopped spinach

2 medium celery stalks

2 medium carrots, peeled

1 medium tomato

1 medium green onion

1 small sprig fresh parsley (optional)

1 cup purified water, divided

1. Place spinach, celery, carrots, tomato, green onion, parsley, and ½ cup water in a blender and blend until thoroughly combined.

2. If necessary, continue adding remaining ½ cup water while blending until desired texture is achieved.

The Power of Parsley

That green garnish on the side of your plate is not given the attention it deserves! This green leafy herb is rich in vitamins and minerals. In just one serving of this cleansing green, there are impressive amounts of vitamins K, C, and A as well as iron and folate. By including just 2 tablespoons parsley in your daily diet, you'll consume more than 153 percent of your needed vitamin K.

Sweet Green Smoothie

Smoothies can be a helpful way to sneak extra vegetables into your day. The mango in this recipe is so sweet and flavorful, you may not even know the spinach is there!

INGREDIENTS | SERVES 1

1 medium banana, frozen

1 cup chopped spinach

1 medium mango, peeled and chopped

2 tablespoons unsweetened applesauce

2 tablespoons water

1 tablespoon ground flaxseed

Add all ingredients to the blender and blend until smooth.

Save the Bananas

If you notice that your banana bunch is starting to get overripe, with a noticeable speckling of brown dots, then now is the time! Simply remove the peel, slice, and freeze. Be sure to package the banana in small serving portions to be used in your smoothie recipes.

Berry Nutty Smoothie

Research has shown that people who eat ¼ cup nuts a day live longer.
That should be enough to convince you to try this smoothie!

INGREDIENTS | SERVES 1

½ cup unsweetened coconut milk

1 medium banana, frozen

1 cup frozen berries

¼ cup walnuts

1 tablespoon ground flaxseed

Add all ingredients to the blender and blend until smooth.

Eat Your Nuts (and Their Skins)

Nuts have a couple of layers: the hard outer shell and a thin skin. It is often tempting to pick off this thin skin, but you should resist doing so because this is the best part of the nut—where the mega source of antioxidants are found.

Green Grape Greatness Smoothie

Hemp and chia seeds provide additional protein and fat to round out the nutritional profile of this sweet smoothie.

INGREDIENTS | SERVES 1

1 cup green grapes

1 medium banana, frozen

1 cup chopped spinach

Juice of 1 medium lime

1 tablespoon shelled hemp seeds

1 teaspoon chia seeds

Add all ingredients to the blender and blend until smooth.

Pear-fect Avocado Smoothie

*Avocado and mango give this smoothie an extra creamy appeal,
not to mention the added antioxidant appeal from the spinach and mango.*

INGREDIENTS | SERVES 2

¼ cup apple juice or water

½ medium avocado

1 cup homemade or unsweetened applesauce

1 medium pear, core removed

1 medium mango, peeled and chopped

1 cup chopped spinach

1 tablespoon shelled hemp seeds

Add all ingredients to the blender and blend until smooth.

Blackberry Blast Smoothie

You can alter this recipe by adding other berries, so how about a Strawberry or Blueberry Blast?

INGREDIENTS | SERVES 2

¼ cup orange juice

1 medium mango, peeled and chopped

1 cup blackberries

1 cup plain, nonfat Greek yogurt

1 tablespoon ground flaxseed

1 tablespoon shelled hemp seeds

Add all ingredients to the blender and blend until smooth.

The Green Go-Getter

Packed with green spinach and apples, this creamy green smoothie will kick off your morning with a boost of essential amino acids, vitamins, minerals, and an absolutely amazing taste.

INGREDIENTS | MAKES 3–4 CUPS

1 cup chopped spinach

2 medium green apples, peeled and cored

1 medium banana

1 cup purified water, divided

1. Place spinach, apples, banana, and ½ cup water in the blender and blend until thoroughly combined.

2. Continue adding remaining ½ cup water while blending until desired texture is achieved.

A Smoothie for Even the Greenest Green Smoothie Maker!

Some people who are new to creating green smoothies can have a hard time enjoying the powerful taste of the greens. The combination of bananas, apples, and spinach with more fruit than greens provides a sweet taste that balances the intensity of the spinach. This smoothie is a great starter for anyone who is turned off by the overpowering taste of greens.

Paradise Greens Smoothie

This delicious blend of coconut and pineapple will send your mind to a tropical place!

INGREDIENTS | SERVES 1

1 cup unsweetened coconut milk

½ cup pineapple chunks

2 tablespoons pineapple juice

1 medium banana

1 cup chopped kale, stems removed

1 tablespoon shelled hemp seeds

1 tablespoon ground flaxseed

Add all ingredients to the blender and blend until smooth.

Go with the Green

A few green vegetables, such as kale, bok choy, and broccoli, are surprisingly great sources of calcium. They aren't as high in calcium as a glass of milk; however, the calcium in these vegetables is more efficiently absorbed by the body. So, in the end, it does compare to the calcium in milk!

Cucumber Lemon Smoothie

This refreshingly sweet smoothie is secretly packed with fiber-, vitamin-, and mineral-rich spinach. In total, it provides at least three servings of fruits and vegetables per smoothie!

INGREDIENTS | SERVES 2

½ medium cucumber, sliced

1 cup homemade or unsweetened applesauce

1 medium banana

2 cups chopped spinach

1 medium mango, peeled and chopped

Juice of 1 medium lemon

2 tablespoons water

Add all ingredients to the blender and blend until smooth.

Savoy Smoothie

The beta carotene in this smoothie will help keep you energized and focused throughout the day. Whether you're looking for a great morning start or a quick and healthy lunch idea, this smoothie is a great go-to!

INGREDIENTS | SERVES 4

1 cup chopped Savoy cabbage

1 medium beet, peeled and chopped

1 medium carrot, peeled and chopped

1 medium apple, cored, peeled, and chopped

1 medium banana

1 cup vanilla almond milk

1. Place cabbage, beet, carrot, apple, banana, and ½ cup almond milk in a blender and blend until thoroughly combined.

2. Add remaining ½ cup almond milk while blending until desired texture is achieved.

Savoy and Vitamin K

Cabbage is packed with vitamin K, whose most well-known benefit is its large responsibility in blood clotting. By consuming just 1 cup chopped Savoy cabbage, you'll be getting more than 90 percent of your recommended daily allowance of vitamin K.

Frozen Breakfast Treat

Substituting soymilk for the coconut milk will increase the protein in this smoothie.

INGREDIENTS | SERVES 2

2 tablespoons almond butter

2 cups unsweetened coconut milk

1 medium banana, frozen

1 tablespoon honey

¼ cup almonds

Add all ingredients to the blender and blend until smooth.

Milk, Milk, and More Milk!

Whether you choose cow, soy, almond, or coconut milk, be sure to check the labels. The two most important things to check are saturated fat and calcium. The lower the amount of saturated fat in the milk, the better. And when it comes to calcium, surprisingly not all milks have the same amount. The label lists calcium as a percentage of the daily value. Try picking a milk that has at least 25 percent of the daily value for calcium; this is equal to 250 milligrams calcium. You may find some brands that have up to 45 percent of the daily value.

CHAPTER 8

Sensational Salads and Staple Dressings

Apple Coleslaw

This coleslaw recipe is a refreshing and sweet alternative to the traditional coleslaw with mayonnaise. Additionally, the sesame seeds give it a nice, nutty flavor.

INGREDIENTS | SERVES 4

2 cups packaged coleslaw mix
1 unpeeled tart apple, chopped
½ cup chopped celery
½ cup chopped green pepper
¼ cup flaxseed oil
2 tablespoons lemon juice
1 teaspoon sesame seeds

1. In a bowl combine the coleslaw mix, apple, celery, and green pepper.

2. In a small bowl, whisk remaining ingredients. Pour over coleslaw and toss to coat.

Seeds versus Nuts

Nuts have a higher omega-6 to omega-3 ratio. Seeds, on the other hand, have a much different profile. Seeds have much lower saturated fat content and are more easily digested by individuals with intestinal issues.

Give Me a Beet

*The creamy combination of goat cheese and avocado topped
with tangy balsamic gives this salad the perfect beet!*

INGREDIENTS | SERVES 4

2 medium beets

1 medium avocado, diced

2 tablespoons goat cheese crumbles

2 tablespoons balsamic vinegar

6 cups arugula

Moving Out of Your Comfort Zone

Beets can be purchased precooked in a can or package, but if you give it a try, you will find that cooking fresh beets is really a piece of cake. Once you prepare your own, going back to canned beets may be difficult. Fresh beets are juicy and naturally full of flavor without all the preservatives of the canned and packaged varieties.

1. Fill a large stockpot with water, place beets in a strainer basket, and cover and cook over medium heat 40 minutes or until beets are easily pierced with a fork. Remove beets from pot to cool. Once you are able to handle them, slip the skin off of the beets and dice into small pieces. Place beets in the refrigerator until cooled and salad is ready to assemble.

2. To assemble the salad, combine beets, avocado, and goat cheese and toss with balsamic vinegar. Serve mixture over a bed of arugula.

Red, White, and Green Salad

You can bulk up this salad into a meal by serving it over a bed of fiber-rich greens.

INGREDIENTS | SERVES 4

6 medium Roma tomatoes, seeded and diced

1 medium avocado, diced

4 ounces mozzarella, cubed

½ tablespoon sea salt

1 tablespoon olive oil

Combine all ingredients in a medium bowl. Chill 30 minutes and serve.

Take It All with a Grain of Salt

Before adding salt to your recipe, be sure to think about the ingredients you are using. If you are choosing fresh or frozen foods that do not contain salt, it may be okay to add a little salt to season your recipe. Canned foods and other processed foods (anything in a package) usually already contain salt, so think twice before adding more when using these ingredients.

Honey Citrus and Avocado Spinach Salad

*The fresh lemon and orange flavors of this salad make it perfect
for any summer day, or winter day—really, any day!*

INGREDIENTS | SERVES 6

8 cups chopped spinach

1 medium red onion, peeled and finely diced

2 medium oranges, peeled, separated, and diced

1 medium avocado, diced

¼ cup feta cheese crumbles

¼–½ cup Honey Lemon Dressing (see recipe in this chapter)

1. In a large salad bowl, combine the spinach, red onion, oranges, avocado, and feta.

2. When ready to serve, toss salad with dressing.

Not the Usual Fruit Salad

Nowadays it is extremely common to mix green vegetables with a variety of fruit to maximize the flavor contrast of sweet and savory. To some, this may seem outrageous! Mixing fruit and vegetables in a salad? If this seems to create a roadblock for you and your taste buds, try this salad. It will help you cross over into the world of vegetable and fruit salads.

Double Roasted Corn and Chickpea Salad

If you are in a hurry, this salad can quickly be thrown together in 10 minutes or less by skipping step number 1 (roasting the corn). This is a perfect staple recipe for any busy weeknight dinner.

INGREDIENTS | SERVES 4

1½ cups frozen corn

2 tablespoons olive oil, divided

1 medium white onion, peeled and diced

1 (15-ounce) can chickpeas, drained and rinsed

8 cups chopped arugula or spinach

2 tablespoons diced red onion

2 sun-dried tomatoes in oil, diced

12 kalamata olives, chopped

1 ounce goat cheese crumbles

4 teaspoons balsamic vinegar

Shortcut Finder

Trader Joe's carries the most flavorful, quick, and easy roasted corn, which has been charbroiled and frozen. This is a quick substitute and timesaver for the actual roasted corn in this recipe but also can be added to a lot of other recipes (pretty much any soup or dish with beans) to enhance the flavor.

1. Preheat oven to 450°F. Toss corn with 1 tablespoon olive oil and arrange in a single layer on a cookie sheet. Bake corn 10 minutes or until golden brown. Remove from oven and allow to cool.

2. In a medium skillet, sauté white onion with 1 tablespoon olive oil over medium heat until caramelized. Add chickpeas to pan and continue to sauté 2–3 minutes, stirring frequently. Remove from heat and allow to cool.

3. Arrange arugula in 4 serving bowls. Top with roasted corn, chickpeas, red onion, sun-dried tomatoes, olives, and goat cheese. Add vinegar and lightly toss to coat.

Watermelon Basil Salad

This is a staple salad for the summer months when watermelons are at their prime.
Add an extra zing with a drizzle of balsamic vinegar.

INGREDIENTS | SERVES 4

4 cups cubed seedless watermelon

2 medium heirloom tomatoes, diced

1 medium cucumber, peeled and diced

¼ cup feta cheese crumbles

1 tablespoon olive oil

¼ cup fresh basil, chopped

¼ teaspoon sea salt

1. Combine watermelon, tomatoes, cucumber, and feta in a medium bowl. Toss lightly with olive oil, basil, and sea salt.

2. Chill at least 1 hour prior to serving.

Triple Green Salad

The flavor blend of savory avocado, kale, and lime with sweet cranberries brings this salad to life for all of your senses.

INGREDIENTS | SERVES 4

1 bunch kale, stemmed and chopped

1 teaspoon sea salt

1 medium avocado, diced

Juice of 1 medium lime

2 teaspoons olive oil

½ cup dried cranberries

1. Place kale in a large bowl. Massage kale leaves with salt for a few minutes to soften.

2. Add remaining ingredients and toss before serving.

Ever-So-Popular Kale

Kale is a glamorized green that has gotten more publicity than ever but actually for very good reason. Kale is one of the most antioxidant-rich foods, and it is very low in calories and carbohydrates. Kale also has fiber, which slows down the absorption of the few carbs it contains. Based on its high fiber content and low calorie content, it can be part of a healthy weight-maintenance or weight-loss diet.

Rainbow Salad with Cashews

This is the most colorful salad you will ever prepare and enjoy!

INGREDIENTS | SERVES 6

12 cups chopped spinach

2 medium mangos, peeled and diced

1 cup blueberries

1 cup diced kiwi

1 cup diced strawberries

1 large avocado, diced

½ medium red onion, peeled and finely diced

½ cup chopped cashews

½ cup The Best Balsamic Dressing (see recipe in this chapter)

1. Fill a large salad bowl with spinach. Top with mangos, blueberries, kiwi, strawberries, avocado, onion, and cashews.

2. Toss salad with dressing just prior to serving.

Avocado Tomato Quinoa Salad

Quinoa (pronounced keen-waa) is a fiber-rich carbohydrate that has a nutty flavor and is a great alternative to plain old white rice.

INGREDIENTS | SERVES 6

2 cups quinoa

4 cups chopped spinach

1 cup diced Roma or heirloom tomatoes

1 large avocado, diced

1 tablespoon olive oil

½ teaspoon sea salt

1. Prepare quinoa according to the package instructions. Allow to cool before assembling salad.

2. In a large salad bowl, mix together quinoa, spinach, tomatoes, and avocado.

3. Drizzle olive oil over the mixture, sprinkle with salt, and toss lightly.

For the Love of Cucumber

If the skin of the cucumber seems to be too much fiber for you, try using a potato peeler to partially skin the cucumber while still getting some of the fiber benefits.

INGREDIENTS | SERVES 4

2 medium cucumbers, diced
½ medium red onion, peeled and diced
½ cup chopped fresh cilantro
½ cup rice vinegar
2 tablespoons sugar

Combine all ingredients in a large bowl, mixing well. Refrigerate at least 1 hour prior to serving.

Sugar versus Splenda

A common goal of the blood sugar diet is to reduce the amount of sugar in your diet. But how do you know if you should use sugar or an artificial sweetener? Most people are able to process small amounts of sugar in their diets without difficulty; it's just when large amounts are eaten or when the body is not working well (as in the case of diabetes) that the artificial sweetener may be helpful. The goal is to keep things as natural as possible, so stevia or sucralose (Splenda) would be the better, more natural substitutes.

Pear and Walnut Salad

Avoid a soggy salad by waiting until serving time to add the dressing. If you feel like there is going to be salad left over, you may want to dress your salad in batches to keep the greens fresh and crisp.

INGREDIENTS | SERVES 4

8 cups chopped spinach

2 medium pears, sliced

½ cup chopped walnuts

½ cup goat cheese crumbles

¼–½ cup The Best Balsamic Dressing (optional) (see recipe in this chapter)

1. In a large bowl, toss together spinach, pears, walnuts, and goat cheese.

2. Just before serving, toss with dressing if desired.

Dare to Go Bare

Challenge your taste buds to enjoy the fresh flavors of your salad by nixing the dressing. This tactic reduces not only calories but also fat. Salads that contain avocado and nuts are able to hold their own with the rich, flavorful fat content. Ingredients such as olives, blue cheese, capers, and sun-dried tomatoes provide such a salty, savory appeal that dressing is really not needed.

Lemon Spinach Orzo Salad

This spinach pasta salad has a unique lemony zip.

INGREDIENTS | SERVES 4

2 cups prepared orzo

4 cups chopped spinach

¼ cup feta cheese

2 tablespoons olive oil

Juice and zest of 1 lemon

¼ teaspoon sea salt

½ teaspoon ground black pepper

1. Prepare orzo according to the package instructions. Allow to cool prior to preparing salad.

2. In a salad bowl, mix orzo, spinach, and feta.

3. In a small bowl, whisk together olive oil, lemon juice and zest, salt, and pepper.

4. Pour dressing over salad, tossing well. Refrigerate at least 30 minutes before serving.

Fruit-Filled Kale Salad

Look for Honeycrisp or Pink Lady apples to give this salad a sweet pop. This is a great way to increase the level of sweetness without having to add sugar.

INGREDIENTS | SERVES 4

8 cups chopped kale

½ cup pomegranate seeds

1 medium apple, cored and diced

½ cup feta cheese

1 medium avocado, diced

½ teaspoon sea salt

½ cup Apple Vinaigrette (see recipe in this chapter)

1. In a large bowl, toss together kale, pomegranate seeds, apple, feta, avocado, and sea salt.

2. Just before serving, toss with dressing.

Mixed Greens Salad with Steak

This salad makes an excellent protein-packed lunch to power you through your afternoon. Try slicing leftover sirloin steak from last night's barbecue to make this a speedy dish.

INGREDIENTS | SERVES 1

1½ cups mixed greens

1 medium green onion, roughly chopped

¼ cup red bell pepper strips

1 medium radish, thinly sliced

¼ cup bean sprouts

3 ounces lean grilled steak, thinly sliced

2 tablespoons The Best Balsamic Dressing (see recipe in this chapter)

1. Place mixed greens on a large plate. Top with chopped green onion, bell pepper strips, radish slices, and bean sprouts.

2. Gently lay steak slices on top of vegetables and drizzle with balsamic dressing. Steak slices can be served hot or cold.

Going for the Greek

The flavors of this salad are so rich and delightful that you may find that the dressing is not necessary.

INGREDIENTS | SERVES 4

8 cups chopped spinach

1 cup chickpeas

½ medium cucumber, diced

½ medium red onion, peeled and diced

2 Roma tomatoes, diced

¼ cup kalamata olives

¼ cup chopped pepperoncini

¼ cup feta cheese crumbles

¼ cup almond slivers

½ cup The Best Balsamic Dressing (optional) (see recipe in this chapter)

1. Fill a large salad bowl with spinach, then layer on the chickpeas, cucumber, onion, tomatoes, olives, pepperoncini, feta, and almonds.

2. Toss salad with dressing just prior to serving if desired.

Mandarin Snap Pea Salad

This unique blend of ingredients creates an unforgettable salad to serve at your next dinner party. Try serving alongside grilled chicken teriyaki for a boost of protein and Asian flavors.

INGREDIENTS | SERVES 8

¾ pound snap peas, cut into ½" pieces

1 cup canned mandarin oranges, drained

1½ cups canned kidney beans, drained and rinsed

1 cup thinly sliced red onion

½ cup chopped fresh parsley

2 cups chopped cabbage

⅓ cup Poppy Seed Dressing (see recipe in this chapter)

1. In medium bowl, combine snap peas, mandarin oranges, kidney beans, onion, parsley, and cabbage.

2. Mix in dressing; refrigerate several hours before serving.

Cashew-Garlic Ranch Dressing

This is a delicious and versatile recipe. Try making it with raw almonds or almond butter if you don't have cashews on hand. If you like extra spice, add an extra teaspoon of chili sauce before mixing.

INGREDIENTS | YIELDS ABOUT ¾ CUP; SERVING SIZE: 1 TABLESPOON

¼ cup raw cashews, or ⅛ cup cashew butter without salt

½ cup water

½ teaspoon stone-ground mustard

1½ tablespoons chili sauce

½ teaspoon horseradish

1 teaspoon Bragg's Liquid Aminos, or tamari sauce

1 clove garlic

1½ teaspoons honey

⅛ teaspoon pepper

1. Process cashews and water in blender or food processor until creamy.

2. Add remaining ingredients; mix well. Refrigerate for 30 minutes.

Honey Lemon Dressing

Homemade dressings are usually good for a few weeks in the refrigerator.
Prepare this one ahead of time and enjoy with a variety of green salads.

INGREDIENTS | MAKES 1 CUP

¼ cup lemon juice

¼ cup honey

½ cup olive oil

¼ teaspoon salt

¼ teaspoon ground black pepper

¼ teaspoon garlic powder

In a small mixing bowl, combine the ingredients and whisk well. Refrigerate until ready to use.

The Perfect Dressing

Once you find a dressing you like, feel free to try mixing and matching salads with that dressing. Simple ingredient swaps, like spices and herbs, will keep you from salad boredom. The flavor possibilities are endless!

The Best Balsamic Dressing

This is the very best balsamic dressing you'll ever taste.
As an added bonus, it'll be ready in just a few minutes!

INGREDIENTS | MAKES 1 CUP

½ cup olive oil

¼ cup balsamic vinegar

1 tablespoon Dijon mustard

1 tablespoon garlic powder

2 teaspoons brown sugar

½ teaspoon sea salt

In a small mixing bowl, combine all ingredients and whisk well to emulsify. Cover and refrigerate until ready to use.

Apple Vinaigrette

Honey and Dijon mustard help emulsify the dressing to keep the oil and vinegar from separating.

INGREDIENTS | MAKES 1½ CUPS

½ cup olive oil

¼ cup apple cider vinegar

1 tablespoon honey

1 tablespoon Dijon mustard

2 tablespoons onion flakes

½ teaspoon sea salt

¼ teaspoon ground black pepper

In a small mixing bowl, combine all ingredients and whisk well. Cover and refrigerate until ready to use.

From Solid to Liquid

One thing that may happen when the dressing is refrigerated is that the oil may slightly solidify. A quick remedy is to simply take the dressing out of the refrigerator and set it near the stove while you are preparing dinner. This will allow the oil to return to its liquid form.

Poppy Seed Dressing

Prepare and store the dressing in a Mason jar; that way, you can shake it up to help the oil and vinegar stay mixed a little longer.

INGREDIENTS | MAKES 1¼ CUPS

½ cup red wine vinegar

¼ cup orange juice

½ cup olive oil

1 teaspoon Splenda Brown Sugar Blend or brown sugar

1 teaspoon dry mustard

1 teaspoon sea salt

1 tablespoon poppy seeds

In a small mixing bowl, combine all ingredients and whisk well. Cover and refrigerate until ready to use.

Bye-Bye, HFCS!

Probably the number-one benefit of making your own dressing is that you can control the ingredients added. Frequently, store-bought dressings have high fructose corn syrup (HFCS), which has been linked to obesity and diabetes.

CHAPTER 9

Soup Lovers

Sweet Potato–Apple Soup

Oven roasting the apples, sweet potatoes, and carrots enriches their natural flavors, making this soup both sweet and savory and one that you are sure to love.

INGREDIENTS | SERVES 6

4 medium sweet potatoes, sliced into ¼" pieces

2 medium red apples, sliced into ¼" pieces

6 medium carrots, peeled and sliced into ¼" pieces

4 tablespoons olive oil, divided

1 medium onion, peeled and sliced

4 cups vegetable or chicken broth

⅛ teaspoon salt

⅛ teaspoon ground black pepper

Chop or Purée, Either Way!

As an alternative, you may chop the sweet potatoes, carrots, and apples into small cubes instead of puréeing to make this soup more like a stew. Or, if you are unsure, purée half and keep the other half chunky—that should satisfy everyone!

1. Preheat oven to 400°F. Toss sweet potatoes, apples, and carrots with 2 tablespoons olive oil and arrange in a single layer on 2 cookie sheets. Roast in oven for 35–40 minutes until lightly browned.

2. Meanwhile, in a large pot, sauté onion in remaining 2 tablespoons olive oil over medium heat until soft, about 5 minutes.

3. Add roasted vegetables, apples, and broth to pot. Bring to a boil, then cover and simmer 15–20 minutes until all ingredients are soft.

4. Carefully purée soup in food processor. Work in batches if necessary.

5. Season with salt and pepper.

Curried Kale and Lentil Stew

This is a no-fuss dinner. Simply fill your pot with the ingredients and your stomach with a flavorful, fiber-rich meal.

INGREDIENTS | SERVES 6

2 tablespoons Smart Balance Buttery Spread

1 medium white onion, peeled and diced

2 cloves garlic, peeled and pressed

3 cups lentils, rinsed

6 cups vegetable or chicken broth

1½ tablespoons curry powder

2 bunches kale, stemmed and chopped

Load Up on Lentils

Lentils are a type of legume that contain an unbelievable amount of blood sugar–stabilizing fiber, nearly 16 grams per cup. By including lentils in your diet, you will not only help prevent diabetes, you will also reduce your risk of common cancers and heart disease.

1. In a large pot, melt buttery spread over medium-low heat. Once melted, add onion and sauté until soft, approximately 4–5 minutes. Then add pressed garlic; sauté 1 minute or until fragrant.

2. Add lentils, broth, and curry powder to pot and increase heat to bring to a boil. Cover and reduce heat to low. Simmer for 45 minutes or until lentils are soft.

3. Add kale to the pot; cover and let cook another 5–10 minutes until softened.

Black Bean Soup

If you can't take the heat, try substituting a seeded, chopped jalapeño pepper or omitting the serrano pepper completely.

INGREDIENTS | SERVES 6

1 medium red onion, peeled and diced

1 medium serrano pepper, seeded and diced

1 tablespoon olive oil

1 medium red bell pepper, seeded and diced

2 cups prepared black beans or 1 (15-ounce) can black beans, drained and rinsed

2 cups corn, roasted

4 cups vegetable broth

3 medium Roma tomatoes, diced

½ cup finely chopped fresh cilantro

2 cups chopped spinach

¼ cup shredded queso fresco (or other cheese)

1 medium avocado, diced

1. In a large pot, sauté onion and serrano pepper in olive oil over medium heat until onion is translucent, about 10 minutes. Then add bell pepper; sauté another 5 minutes.

2. Add beans, corn, and vegetable broth. Bring to a boil, then reduce heat and simmer 10 minutes.

3. Stir in tomatoes, cilantro, and spinach. Cover and remove from heat, allowing spinach to wilt, then serve topped with queso and avocado.

Cold Roasted Red Pepper Soup

Red bell peppers are the star of this meal, but you could try using orange or yellow peppers for a vibrant change. Green bell peppers could work, too, but adjust seasonings to taste, as they aren't as sweet as the red, orange, and yellow varieties.

INGREDIENTS | SERVES 4

1 teaspoon olive oil

½ cup chopped white onion

3 roasted red bell peppers, seeded and chopped (see recipe in sidebar)

3¼ cups low-fat, reduced-sodium chicken broth

½ cup plain, nonfat Greek yogurt

½ teaspoon sea salt (optional)

4 sprigs fresh basil (optional)

1. Heat a large stockpot over medium-high heat. Add olive oil and onion; sauté until onion is transparent, about 5–7 minutes. Add peppers and broth. Bring to a boil; reduce heat and simmer 15 minutes.

2. Remove from heat; purée in blender or food processor until smooth.

3. Allow to cool. Stir in yogurt and salt if desired; chill well in refrigerator. Garnish soup with fresh basil sprigs if desired.

Roasting Red Peppers

The traditional method of roasting a red pepper is to use a long-handled fork to hold the pepper over the open flame of a gas burner until it's charred. Of course, there are a variety of other methods as well. You can place the pepper on a rack set over an electric burner and turn it occasionally, until the skin is blackened. This should take about 4–6 minutes. You can also put the pepper over direct heat on a preheated grill. Use tongs to turn the pepper occasionally. Another method is to broil the pepper on a broiler rack about 2" from the heat, turning the pepper every 5 minutes. Total broiling time will be about 15–20 minutes, until the skin is blistered and charred. The key to peeling the peppers is letting them sit in their steam in a closed container until they are cool. Once the peppers are cool, the skin will rub or peel off easily.

Rosemary Cream of Mushroom Soup

This recipe is a much healthier alternative to the usual canned condensed cream of mushroom soup, which is full of sodium and fat.

INGREDIENTS | SERVES 6

1 medium white onion, peeled and chopped

1 teaspoon olive oil

3 large portabella mushrooms, chopped

1 (10-ounce) package white mushrooms, chopped

3 sprigs fresh rosemary, stems removed, leaves chopped, plus one sprig for garnish

2 cloves garlic, peeled and minced

1 bay leaf

1 tablespoon reduced-sodium soy sauce

1½ tablespoons almond flour

2 cups vegetable broth

2 cups unsweetened almond milk

2 tablespoons freshly grated Parmesan cheese (optional)

2 tablespoons chopped almonds

1. In a large stockpot, sauté onion in olive oil over medium heat until translucent, about 8–10 minutes. Add mushrooms to pan and continue to sauté another 5–7 minutes. Then add rosemary and garlic and continue cooking another 10–12 minutes until mushrooms have changed color and become smaller in size.

2. Add bay leaf and soy sauce to the mushroom mixture and allow to cook another 3–4 minutes.

3. Meanwhile, in a small bowl, mix almond flour into broth and almond milk, then add to soup mixture. Cover and allow soup to simmer over medium-low heat 15–20 minutes, stirring occasionally.

4. Remove bay leaf. Serve sprinkled with Parmesan cheese if desired, almonds, and a rosemary sprig.

Garden Veggie Soup

Pump up this soup into a heartier meal, increasing both fiber and protein, by adding your favorite beans, such as black, butter, or chickpeas.

INGREDIENTS | SERVES 6

1 tablespoon olive oil
¾ cup sliced carrots
½ cup diced white onion
2 cloves garlic, peeled and minced
4 cups broth of choice
1½ cups diced cabbage
½ cup green beans
2 tablespoons tomato paste
1 teaspoon dried basil
¼ teaspoon dried oregano
¼ teaspoon salt
½ cup diced zucchini

1. In a large stockpot, heat olive oil over medium-high heat, add carrots, onion, and garlic, and sauté until softened, approximately 5 minutes.

2. Add broth, cabbage, beans, tomato paste, basil, oregano, and salt. Bring to a boil, then lower heat and simmer uncovered 30 minutes. Add zucchini and continue simmering 5 more minutes before serving.

Weekend Prep = Success!

Weekends can be a great time to get organized, nutritionally speaking, for the week. Meal plan, grocery shop, chop, portion, and store ingredients to save time preparing meals during the busy weekdays.

Garlic White Bean and Kale Soup

This recipes calls for two bunches of kale, but feel free to add even more. Fill the pot with as much kale as possible, cover, and allow to cook down. You can repeat this step as many times as you like for an extra antioxidant boost (vitamins A and C).

INGREDIENTS | SERVES 8

1 medium white onion, peeled and diced

1½ teaspoons olive oil

4 cloves garlic, peeled and finely minced

4 cups vegetable broth

2 (15-ounce) cans white beans, drained and rinsed

2 bunches kale, stemmed and chopped

½ cup feta cheese

Juice of 1 medium lemon

1. In a large stockpot, sauté onion in olive oil over medium heat until translucent, about 5–7 minutes. Add garlic and sauté another 1–2 minutes until fragrant.

2. Add broth and beans; bring to a boil.

3. Fill pot with kale, cover, and remove from heat. Allow kale to cook down for 5 minutes.

4. Serve topped with 1 tablespoon feta cheese and a squeeze of lemon juice.

Sweet Potato Chili

The chipotle pepper in adobo sauce gives this chili some kick.
Try adding more if you like the spice.

INGREDIENTS | SERVES 8

1 medium white onion, peeled and diced

2 tablespoons olive oil

1 pound sweet potatoes, cubed

1 medium red bell pepper, seeded and diced

4 cloves garlic, peeled and finely minced

4 cups vegetable broth

2 cups prepared black beans or 2 (15-ounce) cans black beans, drained and rinsed

1 chipotle pepper in adobo sauce, puréed or minced

6 medium Roma tomatoes, diced

¼ cup plain, nonfat Greek yogurt

1 medium green onion, sliced

1. In a large stockpot, sauté onion in olive oil over medium heat until translucent, about 8–10 minutes. Add sweet potatoes and red pepper, stirring well to cover in oil. Cook about 10 minutes until sweet potatoes and red pepper soften. Add garlic, stirring well to mix in, and cook until fragrant, about 1–2 minutes.

2. Add broth, black beans, chipotle pepper, and tomatoes. Bring to a boil, cover, and simmer 15–20 minutes.

3. Serve topped with a dollop of Greek yogurt and sliced green onion.

Sour Cream Lovers

Sour cream is so delicious when added on top of tacos, chili, and baked potatoes. Unfortunately, your heart is not so impressed with the high saturated fat content. Substituting plain, nonfat Greek yogurt is an amazing way to cut back on the saturated fat and replace it with lean protein—a win-win situation. Give this one a try!

Curried Butternut Squash Soup

Be sure you have a good knife or serrated peeler to cut the thick skin off of the squash. If you are short on time, you may want to purchase the butternut squash already peeled and diced.

INGREDIENTS | SERVES 6

2 pounds butternut squash, peeled and cut into ½" pieces

3 tablespoons olive oil, divided

1 medium white onion, peeled and diced

4 cloves garlic, peeled and pressed

4 cups vegetable broth

2 tablespoons curry powder

½ tablespoon cayenne pepper

¼ cup unsweetened almond milk

2 tablespoons honey

1 tablespoon salt

¼ teaspoon ground black pepper

1. Preheat oven to 400°F. In a medium casserole dish, use your hand to coat butternut squash with 1½ tablespoons olive oil. Bake in the oven for 30 minutes or until squash is soft and lightly browned.

2. Meanwhile, in a large stockpot over medium heat, sauté onion with remaining 1½ tablespoons olive oil until translucent, about 5–7 minutes. Then add garlic; sauté an additional 1–2 minutes until fragrant.

3. Add butternut squash, broth, curry powder, and cayenne pepper to pot. Bring to a boil, then cover and simmer 15–20 minutes.

4. Remove from heat. Add almond milk and honey to mixture, then purée until smooth. Taste and season as preferred with additional curry powder, salt, and pepper.

Lentil Vegetable Soup

This low-maintenance recipe is perfect for nights when you don't have a lot of energy to cook. After you prep your vegetables, the soup practically cooks itself!

INGREDIENTS | SERVES 4

5 cups water or your choice of broth

1 medium sweet potato, peeled and chopped

1 cup lentils

2 medium white onions, peeled and chopped

¼ cup barley

2 tablespoons dried parsley

2 medium carrots, peeled and sliced

1 celery stalk, chopped

2 teaspoons cumin

Combine all ingredients in stockpot; simmer until lentils are soft, about 1 hour.

Roasted Sweet Potatoes and Cauliflower Soup

This soup is delicious served hot or cold, and is even better the next day.

INGREDIENTS | SERVES 8

1 head cauliflower, outer stems removed, chopped into small florets

4 medium sweet potatoes, peeled and diced

3 tablespoons olive oil, divided

1 teaspoon smoked paprika

½ teaspoon salt

2 teaspoons garlic powder

1 medium white onion, peeled and diced

4 cups vegetable broth

¼ cup sun-dried tomatoes, chopped

C Is for Cruciferous

Cauliflower is a cruciferous vegetable, much like broccoli, kale, Brussels sprouts, arugula, and cabbage, all rich in the (disease-fighting) antioxidant vitamin C. Try to include five servings of cruciferous vegetables in your weekly meals.

1. Preheat oven to 400°F. Place cauliflower and sweet potatoes on cookie sheets and, using hands, coat with 2 tablespoons olive oil. Sprinkle with smoked paprika, salt, and garlic powder. Bake until softened and browned, approximately 10–15 minutes.

2. Meanwhile, in a large stockpot, sauté onion over medium-high heat in remaining 1 tablespoon olive oil until translucent, about 8 minutes.

3. Add vegetable broth and roasted vegetables to pot. Bring to a boil, then reduce heat to low, cover, and simmer 15 minutes.

4. Once cooled, purée soup in food processor. Top with sun-dried tomatoes and serve.

Honey Cinnamon Pumpkin Soup

This sweet and savory soup is a fall harvest favorite. Serve with a large spinach salad, topped with chopped apples, walnuts, and The Best Balsamic Dressing (Chapter 8).

INGREDIENTS | SERVES 6

1 medium white onion, peeled and diced

4 medium apples, cored and diced

4 cloves garlic, peeled and pressed

1 teaspoon olive oil

¼ cup water

1 (15-ounce) can pumpkin

4 cups vegetable broth

½ teaspoon cinnamon

½ teaspoon honey

1. In a medium saucepan, sauté onion, apples, and garlic in olive oil over medium-high heat 3–4 minutes. Add water, bring to a boil, then cover and simmer approximately 8 minutes until soft. Remove from heat and allow to cool, then purée mixture.

2. In a large pot over medium-low heat, combine apple mixture, pumpkin, broth, and cinnamon. Cover and cook 10–15 minutes. Drizzle with honey and serve.

CHAPTER 10

Variety of Veggies

Balsamic Brussels

Never say never! Some people have sworn off Brussels sprouts,
but this recipe may have you rethinking that decision.

INGREDIENTS | SERVES 4

1 medium red onion, peeled and diced

4 tablespoons olive oil, divided

4 cups quartered Brussels sprouts

1 tablespoon balsamic vinegar

1 tablespoon Dijon mustard

1 teaspoon garlic powder

Benefits of Brussels

Even if you hated them as a kid, you should try Brussels sprouts again! Brussels sprouts are among the superfoods that help your body fight off the bad things that can cause cancer or diabetes. Other than the antioxidant load, Brussels sprouts also contain soluble fiber, which helps lower cholesterol.

1. In a medium saucepan, sauté onion in 2 tablespoons olive oil over medium heat. Stir onion frequently until browned, approximately 5–10 minutes.

2. Add Brussels sprouts to pan and stir occasionally until soft and caramelized, about 10–15 minutes.

3. Meanwhile, in a small bowl, whisk together remaining 2 tablespoons olive oil with vinegar, mustard, and garlic powder. Pour over Brussels sprouts and cook 1 additional minute.

Quick-Roasted Carrots

A bag of whole carrots is much easier on the pocketbook than a bag of baby carrots. Either way, these carrots will need to be sliced into smaller sticks to roast quickly.

INGREDIENTS | SERVES 4

1 pound carrots, peeled and cut into thin sticks

1 tablespoon olive oil

½ teaspoon sea salt

1 tablespoon garlic powder

1. Preheat oven to 400°F. Arrange carrots in a single layer on a cookie sheet, then drizzle with olive oil, using hands to toss and coat carrots evenly.

2. Sprinkle with salt and garlic powder. Bake 20–25 minutes until soft and lightly browned. Shake pan halfway through to turn carrots.

Roasted Garlic Cabbage

This cabbage recipe provides a quick and delicious garlicky side for any meal.

INGREDIENTS | SERVES 4

1 head cabbage, sliced into ¼"-thick round pieces

1 tablespoon olive oil

4–6 cloves garlic, peeled and pressed

½ teaspoon sea salt

¼ cup feta cheese

1. Preheat oven to 400°F.

2. Place cabbage rounds on cookie sheet. Using your hands, rub each round with oil. Top with garlic and sprinkle with salt.

3. Bake 20–25 minutes until lightly browned. Top with feta cheese and serve.

Cinnamon Sweet Potatoes

The fiber-rich and sweet-tasting apples and apricots give this sweet potato casserole a unique edge, perfect for your next holiday gathering.

INGREDIENTS | SERVES 6

4 medium sweet potatoes, sliced into ⅛"-thick circles

2 medium apples, cored and thinly sliced

¼ cup diced dried apricots

Juice of 1 medium lemon

⅓ cup honey

½ cup apple cider

1 teaspoon cinnamon

½ cup chopped walnuts

Choose Healthier

There are many alternatives to the traditional sweet potato casseroles, so look for one with a healthier spin. The traditional sweet potato casserole may contain up to 500 calories per serving. That should be enough to steer you away. When choosing a sweet potato casserole replacement, look for a recipe like this one that is not full of sugar, marshmallows, and butter.

1. Preheat oven to 400°F. Spray an 8" × 12" baking dish with cooking spray.

2. Layer sweet potato slices, then apple slices, repeating until both apples and sweet potatoes are arranged. Top with apricots.

3. In a small mixing bowl, whisk together lemon juice, honey, apple cider, and cinnamon. Pour the mixture over the potatoes.

4. Cover with foil and bake 35–40 minutes, then remove foil, top with walnuts, and bake an additional 10–15 minutes until potatoes are soft and lightly browned. Remove from oven and cool 10 minutes before serving.

Extra Crispy Broccoli Florets

This is simply the best way to cook broccoli, hands down. When arranging the broccoli florets on the baking sheet, try placing them stem-side up. This will allow the florets to get crispy and the stems to soften.

INGREDIENTS | SERVES 4

4 cups small broccoli florets
2 teaspoons olive oil
1 tablespoon garlic powder
1½ teaspoons sea salt

No Excuses Here!

Oftentimes, serving a healthy meal seems too time-consuming. Here's the quick and easy solution to your busy night: Pre-chop or purchase chopped broccoli, then just quickly toss and bake, and you'll have a cruciferous veggie to serve hot out of the oven. Adding broccoli or other veggies to your meal may result in weight loss by replacing additional servings of other higher-calorie foods.

1. Preheat oven to 400°F.

2. Toss broccoli florets with olive oil, garlic powder, and salt. Spread in a single layer on a baking sheet.

3. Bake 10–15 minutes until florets become crispy and lightly browned.

4. Allow to cool a few minutes before serving.

Mushrooms and Leeks

Venture out of your comfort zone and purchase some leeks.
You won't be disappointed by the flavor or the ease.

INGREDIENTS | SERVES 4

12 ounces portabella mushrooms, chopped

1 medium zucchini, diced

2 medium leeks, white and light green portions chopped thinly, roots and dark green portions removed

2 tablespoons olive oil

1 clove garlic, peeled and minced

1. In a large skillet, sauté mushrooms, zucchini, and leeks in olive oil over medium heat approximately 20 minutes.

2. Add garlic; continue cooking another 3–5 minutes. Serve hot.

What Exactly Are Leeks?

Leeks are flying under the radar as far as popularity, but as far as onions are concerned, leeks are the king of them all. Leeks have similar health benefits as garlic and onions, most notably the antioxidants that keep your heart healthy. Just be sure to give leeks a thorough wash, as they can harbor quite a bit of dirt between their layers.

Sweet and Spicy Baked Sweet Potato Coins

For a special treat, skip the honey and top sweet potato rounds
with a sprinkle of blue cheese and sliced green onion.

INGREDIENTS | SERVES 4

2 medium sweet potatoes, sliced into
⅛"-thick circles

2 teaspoons olive oil

½ teaspoon sea salt

1 teaspoon garlic powder

½ teaspoon cayenne pepper (optional)

1 teaspoon honey (optional)

1. Preheat oven to 400°F. Lay sweet potatoes in a single layer on a baking sheet, drizzle with olive oil, and toss with hands to coat potatoes evenly. Season potatoes with salt, garlic powder, and cayenne if desired.

2. Bake for 20–25 minutes until lightly browned. Remove from oven and allow to cool for 5 minutes. Drizzle with honey if desired.

Sweet Potatoes versus Yams

Most people think of sweet potatoes and yams as one and the same, but in actuality, that is wrong! Sweet potatoes and yams are just two of the hundreds of types of potatoes. Sweet potatoes are usually the red- to orange-fleshed potatoes, while yams tend to be whiter in color. Because of this difference, yams are lower in beta carotene, a precursor to the antioxidant action of vitamin A.

Vegetable Curry

Serve this fiber-rich veggie dish with a side of white or brown rice, or just enjoy it served solo.

INGREDIENTS | SERVES 6

2 tablespoons olive oil

1 medium white onion, peeled and diced

1 medium sweet potato, diced

1 medium green bell pepper, seeded and diced

1 medium red bell pepper, seeded and diced

½ medium eggplant, diced

1 cup broccoli florets, chopped into small pieces

1 medium zucchini squash, diced

1 small (11-ounce) jar yellow curry sauce

1. In a large saucepan, heat olive oil over medium heat. Add onions, sauté for 3–5 minutes, and then add the rest of the vegetables and cover.

2. Stirring frequently, cook 15–20 minutes until vegetables are softened and lightly browned.

3. Add curry sauce and simmer on low approximately 10 minutes.

Ingredient Finder

Trader Joe's Thai Yellow Curry Sauce is the best sauce around. The important thing to remember is that a little curry sauce goes a long way. If you want to spice it up, add a little red chili sauce or Sriracha.

Fresh Roasted Green Beans

There is really no excuse not to have veggies with dinner. You can throw these beans in the oven and voilà—done in 15 minutes!

INGREDIENTS | SERVES 6

1 pound fresh green beans, ends trimmed
3 teaspoons olive oil
1 teaspoon sea salt
½ teaspoon garlic powder
½ teaspoon onion powder

1. Preheat oven to 400°F.

2. Arrange green beans in a single layer on a baking sheet. Dress with olive oil, salt, garlic powder, and onion powder.

3. Bake 15–20 minutes, stirring halfway through cooking time.

Avocado and Shiitake Pot Stickers

Once you try these California-fusion pot stickers, you'll wish you had made a double batch! These little dumplings don't need to be enhanced with a complex dipping sauce, so serve them plain or with soy sauce.

INGREDIENTS | MAKES 12–15 POT STICKERS

1 medium avocado, diced small

½ cup diced shiitake mushrooms

½ (14-ounce) block silken tofu, crumbled

1 clove garlic, peeled and minced

2 teaspoons balsamic vinegar

1 teaspoon soy sauce

12–15 vegan dumpling wrappers

Water for steaming or oil for pan-frying

Whether Steamed or Fried . . .

In dumpling houses across East Asia, dumplings are served with a little bowl of freshly grated ginger, and diners create a simple dipping sauce from the various condiments on the table. To try it, pour some rice vinegar and a touch of soy sauce over a bit of ginger and add hot chili oil to taste.

1. In a small bowl, gently mash together avocado, mushrooms, tofu, garlic, balsamic vinegar, and soy sauce just until mixed and crumbly.

2. Place about 1½ teaspoons of the filling in the middle of each wrapper. Fold in half and pinch closed, forming little pleats. You may want to dip your fingertips in water to help the dumplings stay sealed if needed.

3. To pan-fry: Heat a thin layer of oil in a large skillet. Carefully add dumplings and cook for just 1 minute. Add about ½ cup water, cover, and cook 3–4 minutes.

4. To steam: Carefully place a layer of dumplings in a steamer, being sure the dumplings don't touch. Place steamer above boiling water and allow to cook, covered, 3–4 minutes.

Roasted Green Chilies

Roasting green chilies may seem like an intimidating feat, but honestly, it doesn't get easier than this. Anaheim chilies are a milder chili, while pasilla chilies will turn up the heat of any of your favorite dishes.

INGREDIENTS | SERVES 8

4 green chilies (Anaheim or pasilla)

Freeze for Later

Another timesaving tactic is to prepare a few peppers at a time, use what you need, then freeze the remainder. Once the peppers have cooled, chop or slice into desired portions, package, and freeze for later use.

1. Preheat broiler. Place chilies on a baking sheet lined with foil.

2. Broil 10 minutes or until skins begin to blacken. Using tongs, flip chilies to the other side and continue to broil another 5–7 minutes until blackened. Remove from broiler.

3. Take chilies off pan and place in a heat-safe bowl with a lid to steam chilies.

4. After 20 minutes, remove chilies from bowl. Using your hands, peel off the outer skin and remove the stems and seeds of chilies.

5. Refrigerate or freeze chilies until ready to use.

Double Cheese Sweet Potato Latkes

These savory potato pancakes are loaded with vitamin A and, more importantly, cheesy goodness.

INGREDIENTS | SERVES 6

1 medium red onion, peeled and diced

4 medium sweet potatoes, grated

½ cup shredded Cheddar cheese

½ cup shredded carrots

1 large egg, beaten

½ cup feta cheese

2 cloves garlic, peeled and pressed

1 teaspoon salt

1 teaspoon garlic salt

¼ cup olive oil

2 tablespoons plain, nonfat Greek yogurt (optional)

½ cup diced green onion

1. Combine onion, sweet potatoes, cheese, carrots, egg, feta, garlic, salt, and garlic salt in a large bowl, mixing well.

2. Heat a medium skillet over medium heat. Coat pan with thin layer of olive oil.

3. Form sweet potato mixture into small patties and cook over medium heat 5–8 minutes; flip and cook another 4–5 minutes until lightly browned. Serve with a dollop of Greek yogurt, if desired, and a sprinkle of green onion.

Zesty Chili Corn on the Cob

If the busy week puts you in a time crunch, simply skip the grill and boil the ears of corn, then season with the chili sauce.

INGREDIENTS | SERVES 4

2 ears corn

1 tablespoon Smart Balance Buttery Spread, melted

1 teaspoon red chili sauce or Sriracha

¼ teaspoon sea salt

Juice of 1 medium lime

Corn on the Carb?

While corn is truly a vegetable, in reality it may be closer to a carbohydrate in the way it works in the body. Corn can be incorporated into the blood sugar diet if you think of it more as a carb and balance it out with additional vegetables and lean proteins.

1. Preheat grill to medium heat and place corn on grill. Cook corn until soft and lightly browned, approximately 10–15 minutes.

2. Meanwhile, mix melted buttery spread with chili sauce in a small bowl.

3. Once corn is removed from grill, spread each ear with buttery sauce, salt, and lime juice.

Marinated Roasted Peppers and Eggplant

Red peppers and eggplant are a classic combination, but other vegetable combinations are great, too. Try adding sliced zucchini, tomatoes, or mushrooms for extra flavor and nutrition.

INGREDIENTS | SERVES 4

1 pound medium red bell peppers

1 large eggplant, sliced into ¼"-thick rounds

4 tablespoons olive oil, divided

1 tablespoon balsamic vinegar

1 tablespoon finely chopped red onion

1 teaspoon dried oregano

¼ teaspoon freshly ground black pepper

1. Follow procedure for roasting red peppers (see sidebar for Cold Roasted Red Pepper Soup in Chapter 9). Set aside.

2. Brush eggplant slices with 2 tablespoons olive oil; place on grill. Grill about 5 minutes on each side until softened. Remove from grill and place in container. Add roasted peppers to container.

3. Prepare marinade by whisking together remaining 2 tablespoons olive oil, balsamic vinegar, onion, oregano, and black pepper; pour over vegetables. Cover and refrigerate for at least 30 minutes.

Mashed Cauliflower

Try not to fool yourself into thinking this will taste exactly like mashed potatoes. That would be setting your taste buds up for disappointment. Enjoy the cauliflower for what it is: a healthy alternative to carb- and fat-loaded mashed potatoes.

INGREDIENTS | SERVES 4

Florets from 1 head cauliflower

2 cloves garlic, peeled

1 tablespoon Smart Balance Buttery Spread

¼ cup feta cheese

¼ cup shredded Cheddar cheese

¼ teaspoon sea salt

¼ teaspoon ground black pepper

1. In a medium pot, boil water, add cauliflower and garlic, then return to a boil and cook 10 minutes.

2. Transfer cauliflower, garlic, and remaining ingredients to a food processor and blend until desired consistency is reached.

What about This or That?

When it comes to choosing healthy alternatives, oftentimes you may get hung up on the ingredients and "the rules." For example, some may say, "What about the two types of cheeses you are adding in this recipe?" Well, it is important to take a step back and think about what else you are and are not using. With this recipe, you are skipping out on the carb load of potatoes and the usual fat load of butter and sour cream, so a little cheese is still a better alternative.

Broccoli Raab with Pine Nuts

Broccoli raab, a pungent, bitter green often used in Italian cooking, is growing in popularity in the United States. Be sure to follow blanching instructions carefully to reduce bitterness.

INGREDIENTS | SERVES 4

¾ pound broccoli raab

1 tablespoon olive oil

4 cloves garlic, peeled and chopped

¼ cup sun-dried tomatoes, chopped

2 tablespoons pine nuts

¼ teaspoon salt

¼ teaspoon red pepper flakes

Preventing Bitter Broccoli Raab

Broccoli raab and other leafy greens such as mustard and collard greens can have a bitter taste once cooked. Rather than add extra salt to offset the bitterness, this recipe calls for blanching 2 minutes, which helps reduce bitterness. Blanching should be done as quickly as possible by starting with water at a full rolling boil, then removing the greens after 2 minutes of boiling. If allowed to cook too long, the boiling process will reduce the amount of water-soluble nutrients found in the vegetables.

1. Prepare and blanch broccoli raab before beginning recipe: Rinse well and trim stems. Loosely chop leafy parts, then blanch in 2 quarts boiling water 2 minutes. Drain well.

2. Heat olive oil in a large skillet; add garlic. Sauté garlic 1–2 minutes; add blanched broccoli raab. Toss together garlic and broccoli raab so that oil and garlic are mixed evenly.

3. Add remaining ingredients; cook additional 2–3 minutes until broccoli raab is tender.

Winter Vegetable Casserole

This incredible casserole is hearty enough to serve as a standalone vegetarian dish.
It also works nicely as a side dish for Thanksgiving dinner.

INGREDIENTS | SERVES 6

3 tablespoons butter

3 tablespoons all-purpose flour

½ teaspoon salt

¼ teaspoon ground white pepper

1½ cups low-fat milk or milk substitute

1½ medium white potatoes, thinly sliced

1½ medium sweet potatoes, thinly sliced

1 cup peeled, sliced parsnips

1 cup sliced turnips

½ cup chopped white onion

1. Preheat oven to 350°F. Spray a 2-quart casserole dish with cooking spray.

2. In a small saucepan over low heat, melt butter; add flour, salt, and pepper to make a roux. Gradually stir in milk with a wire whisk.

3. Bring to a boil, stirring constantly, until milk mixture has thickened into a sauce, about 10 minutes. Remove from heat.

4. Arrange ½ of sliced vegetables in casserole dish; top with ½ of chopped onion and white sauce; repeat to make second layer. Cover and cook in preheated oven for 45 minutes. Uncover and continue to cook until all vegetables are tender, about 60–70 minutes.

5. Let casserole stand 10 minutes before serving.

Potato Medley with Roasted Green Chilies

*You can use any leftover potatoes from this recipe to make potato tacos;
just substitute potatoes where you would usually add the meat.*

INGREDIENTS | SERVES 6

1 medium white onion, peeled and diced

1 medium red bell pepper, seeded and diced

¼ cup olive oil

2 medium sweet potatoes, diced

3 medium white potatoes, diced

2 medium Roma tomatoes, seeded and diced

2 roasted green chilies, diced

½ teaspoon salt

1 teaspoon garlic powder

1 medium avocado, diced

2 tablespoons green salsa (optional)

2 tablespoons shredded pepper jack or Mexican blend cheese (optional)

1. In a large saucepan, sauté onion and red pepper in olive oil over medium heat until softened, approximately 5 minutes.

2. Add potatoes to saucepan. Over medium-low heat, cook 20 minutes or more, stirring often, until potatoes are soft and lightly browned.

3. Add tomatoes and green chilies, cover, and cook an additional 1–2 minutes. Season with salt and garlic powder.

4. Serve with avocado, green salsa, and shredded cheese if desired.

Spinach-Stuffed Mushrooms

There is nothing better than mushrooms on the grill. No, wait!
Actually, there is nothing better than stuffed mushrooms on the grill!

INGREDIENTS | SERVES 4

½ cup feta cheese
1 cup finely chopped spinach
½ cup finely chopped fresh cilantro
½ teaspoon salt
¼ teaspoon ground black pepper
8 medium portabella mushrooms, stems removed

1. In a small bowl, combine all ingredients except mushrooms.

2. Lay 8 mushroom caps stem-side up on a piece of foil. Stuff each cap with mixture. Enclose mushrooms in foil.

3. Place on heated barbecue grill, cooking approximately 10 minutes or until mushrooms and filling are cooked.

CHAPTER 11

Beans and Legumes

Onion Roasted Chickpeas

These chickpeas can be a standalone side or a filling in a pita pocket with the added Greek fixings of spinach, pepperoncini, cucumbers, tomatoes, kalamata olives, and feta.

INGREDIENTS | SERVES 4

1 medium red onion, peeled and finely diced

3 medium green onions, chopped

2 tablespoons olive oil

1 (15-ounce) can chickpeas, drained and rinsed

½ teaspoon sea salt

1 tablespoon garlic powder

1. In a medium saucepan, sauté red and green onions in olive oil over medium-high heat until lightly browned, about 5–7 minutes.

2. Add chickpeas and sauté 2–4 minutes.

3. Season with salt and garlic powder and serve.

Bunless Black Bean Quinoa Burger

Try this patty with a variety of toppings such as a sprinkle of cheese, roasted green chilies, sliced tomato, avocado, sautéed spinach, or any other topping you like. This high-fiber, low-fat burger will definitely fulfill that hamburger craving!

INGREDIENTS | SERVES 8

1 teaspoon olive oil

½ medium white onion, peeled and finely diced

1 teaspoon reduced-sodium soy sauce

2 cloves garlic, peeled and pressed

2 cups cooked quinoa

1 cup prepared black beans

1 cup prepared black beans, puréed

¼ cup ground flaxseed

1 teaspoon ground mustard

¼ teaspoon smoked paprika

1½ teaspoons sea salt

1 teaspoon shredded Cheddar cheese (optional)

1 large avocado, sliced

2 medium Roma tomatoes, sliced

4 teaspoons Dijon mustard

1. In a small skillet, heat olive oil over medium heat. Add onion and sauté slowly 7–10 minutes. Add soy sauce and garlic and continue to cook 1–2 minutes.

2. Meanwhile, in a medium bowl, combine quinoa, black beans, puréed black beans, and flaxseed, mixing well. Season with ground mustard, smoked paprika, and salt.

3. Form mixture into patties. Spray skillet with cooking spray or a small amount of olive oil and cook patties over medium heat for 5 minutes. Flip patties and cook another 2–3 minutes. Top with shredded cheese if desired.

4. Remove from heat. Serve your bunless burger with avocado slices, tomato slices, and Dijon mustard.

Household Staples

It is common to peruse recipes and decide to make or not to make based on the amount of ingredients required. Although this recipe seems to have a laundry list of ingredients, they are all foods that should be staples in your health-driven diet—and are used in many of the other recipes in this book. So start stocking that pantry and refrigerator with lots of beans and fresh vegetables!

Italian White Beans and Rice

This is a quick, inexpensive, and hearty meal that will quickly become a favorite standby on busy nights. It's nutritious, filling, and can easily be doubled for a crowd.

INGREDIENTS | SERVES 4

½ medium onion, diced

2 medium celery stalks, diced

3 cloves garlic, minced

2 tablespoons olive oil

1 (12-ounce) can diced or crushed tomatoes

1 (15-ounce) can cannellini or great northern beans, drained and rinsed

½ teaspoon parsley

½ teaspoon basil

1 cup rice, cooked

1 tablespoon balsamic vinegar

1. In a large skillet, sauté onion, celery, and garlic in olive oil for 3–5 minutes until onion and celery are soft.

2. Reduce heat to medium-low and add tomatoes, beans, parsley, and basil. Cover and simmer for 10 minutes, stirring occasionally.

3. Stir in cooked rice and balsamic vinegar and cook, uncovered, for a few more minutes until liquid is absorbed.

Sun-Dried Tomato Chickpea Roll-Up

*Prepare this wrap for dinner and, while you are at it,
double up and make another wrap for tomorrow's lunch.*

INGREDIENTS | SERVES 1

1 high-fiber tortilla

2 tablespoons hummus

¼ cup canned chickpeas, drained and rinsed

2 tablespoons chopped spinach

2 tablespoons diced cucumber

1 tablespoon chopped sun-dried tomato

1 teaspoon feta cheese

Place tortilla on a plate and spread evenly with hummus. Arrange all ingredients inside and roll up.

Chickpeas or Garbanzo Beans?

The terms *chickpeas* and *garbanzo beans* are often used interchangeably—that's because they are the same thing. Whichever name you prefer, you are referring to a hearty legume, rich in both fiber and protein as well as some key vitamins and minerals that a meat-free diet may be lacking (vitamin B_6, thiamine, iron, phosphorus, magnesium, and zinc).

Mexi-Cali Layered "Lasagna"

This is not your traditional Italian layered lasagna. High-fiber beans, vegetables, and tortillas are sure to please your next dinner crowd on Cinco de Mayo or any night.

INGREDIENTS | SERVES 12

1 medium red onion, peeled and diced

1 medium serrano pepper, seeded and diced

1 medium red bell pepper, seeded and diced

1 tablespoon olive oil

1 cup frozen roasted corn

2 cups spinach, chopped

1 can refried beans or 2 cups puréed pinto beans

½ cup salsa, divided

½ cup shredded Mexican cheese blend, divided

12 small corn tortillas

2 medium green onions, sliced

1. Preheat oven to 375°F.

2. In a medium saucepan, sauté onion, serrano pepper, and red pepper in olive oil over medium-high heat until soft and lightly browned, about 5–7 minutes. Add corn and spinach, heating 5 minutes or until heated and spinach has cooked down.

3. Meanwhile, in a small saucepan, heat refried beans over medium heat stirring frequently.

4. Spread ¼ cup salsa and ¼ cup cheese evenly across the bottom of a medium casserole dish. Then layer 5 corn tortillas. Top with ½ of refried beans, then ½ of vegetable mixture. Repeat with another 5 corn tortillas, remaining refried beans, and then remaining vegetable mixture. Then top with remaining salsa, remaining cheese, and green onions. Bake in oven approximately 15–20 minutes until cheese is melted and lightly browned.

Black and Green Veggie Burritos

Black bean burritos filled with zucchini or yellow summer squash. Just add in the fixings—salsa, avocado slices, and a small dollop of sour cream—the works!

INGREDIENTS | SERVES 4

1 medium white onion, peeled and chopped

2 medium zucchini or yellow squash, cut into thin strips

1 medium bell pepper, any color, seeded and chopped

2 tablespoons olive oil

½ teaspoon dried oregano

½ teaspoon cumin

1 (15-ounce) can black beans, drained and rinsed

1 (4-ounce) can green chilies

1 cup cooked rice

4 large high-fiber tortillas, warmed

1. Heat onion, zucchini, and bell pepper in olive oil over medium-high heat until vegetables are soft, about 4–5 minutes.

2. Reduce heat to low and add oregano, cumin, black beans, and chilies, combining well. Cook, stirring, until heated through.

3. Place ¼ cup rice in the center of each flour tortilla and top with the bean mixture. Fold the bottom of the tortilla up, then snugly wrap one side, then the other.

4. Serve as is, or bake in a 350°F oven 15 minutes for a crispy burrito.

White Bean Salad

A lemony fresh salad with seriously simple prep.
The hardest part is waiting the full 30 minutes before eating!

INGREDIENTS | SERVES 4

1 (15-ounce) can white beans (cannellini or great northern beans), drained and rinsed

½ medium red onion, peeled and diced

Juice of 1 medium lemon

½ cup finely chopped fresh parsley

2 tablespoons olive oil

½ teaspoon sea salt

1 tablespoon garlic powder

In a medium bowl, mix together all ingredients. Refrigerate 30 minutes prior to serving.

The Ever-So-Versatile Bean

Beans provide a good source of protein, iron, and zinc similar to animal proteins (meats), but they also contain high amounts of fiber and other vitamins and minerals similar to vegetables. You could also consider beans a carbohydrate source, as they are rich in complex carbs and, again, ever-so-famous fiber.

Black Bean and Butternut Squash Chili

Squash is an excellent addition to vegetarian chili in this southwestern-style dish.

INGREDIENTS | SERVES 4

1 medium white onion, peeled and chopped

3 cloves garlic, peeled and minced

2 tablespoons oil

1 medium butternut squash, peeled and chopped into chunks

2 (15-ounce) cans black beans, drained and rinsed

1 (28-ounce) can stewed or diced tomatoes, undrained

¾ cup water or vegetable broth

1 tablespoon chili powder

1 teaspoon cumin

¼ teaspoon cayenne pepper

½ teaspoon salt

2 tablespoons chopped fresh cilantro (optional)

1. In a large stockpot over medium-high heat, sauté onion and garlic in oil until soft, about 4 minutes.

2. Reduce heat to medium and add remaining ingredients except cilantro.

3. Cover and simmer 25 minutes. Uncover and simmer another 5 minutes. Top with fresh cilantro just before serving.

Avocado Bean Orzo

This dish contains the perfect balance of protein, fat, and carbohydrates. Increase the portion for a main dish or serve a smaller portion for a side dish; either way, your blood sugar should remain stable.

INGREDIENTS | SERVES 4

1 (15-ounce) can chickpeas, drained and rinsed

2 cups cooked orzo

1 medium avocado, diced

½ medium red onion, peeled and diced

½ cup feta cheese crumbles

Juice of ½ medium lemon

1 tablespoon lemon zest

½ teaspoon sea salt

In a medium bowl, mix together all ingredients. Refrigerate at least 30 minutes before serving.

Kale and White Bean Quesadilla

This fiber-filled dinner is ready in less than 10 minutes!

INGREDIENTS | SERVES 1

¼ medium white onion, peeled and diced

1 teaspoon olive oil

¼ cup chopped kale

¼ cup canned white beans, drained and rinsed

1 high-fiber tortilla

2 tablespoons shredded mozzarella

1 medium Roma tomato, diced

1. In a medium skillet, sauté onion in olive oil over medium heat. After 5 minutes, add kale and white beans, heating an additional 5 minutes until kale cooks down. Remove all ingredients from skillet and place in a bowl.

2. Rinse and dry skillet, then heat skillet over medium heat. Place tortilla in skillet. Next, layer in bean and kale mixture, mozzarella, and tomato. Cook another 4–5 minutes until cheese has melted. Fold in half and remove from heat.

Leftover Lentil Salad

Whenever you are cooking up lentils, be sure to throw in some extra lentils to be used in this easy leftover salad.

INGREDIENTS | SERVES 4

2 cups cooked green lentils

1 tablespoon capers

2 tablespoons diced sun-dried tomatoes

1 cup chopped spinach

In a medium bowl, mix together all ingredients. Refrigerate at least 30 minutes before serving.

Black-Eyed Pea Salad

Because black-eyed peas swell up when they are cooked, many people eat them on New Year's Day to symbolize prosperity and increased wealth.

INGREDIENTS | SERVES 4

1 (15-ounce) can black-eyed peas, drained and rinsed

1 medium avocado, diced

1 cup roasted corn

½ medium red onion, peeled and diced

1 teaspoon ground black pepper

1 tablespoon olive oil

Juice of ½ medium lemon

2 tablespoons shelled hemp seeds

In a medium bowl, mix together all ingredients. Refrigerate at least 30 minutes before serving.

Pumpkin and Lentil Curry

Red lentils complement the pumpkin and coconut best in this salty, sweet curry, but any kind you have on hand will do. Look for frozen chopped squash to cut the preparation time.

INGREDIENTS | SERVES 3

1 medium yellow onion, peeled and chopped

2 cups chopped pumpkin or butternut squash

2 tablespoons olive oil

1 tablespoon curry powder

1 teaspoon cumin

2 small red chilies, minced, or ½ teaspoon red pepper flakes

2 whole cloves

3 cups water or vegetable broth

1 cup lentils

2 medium tomatoes, chopped

8–10 green beans, trimmed and chopped

¾ cup unsweetened coconut milk

1. In a medium stockpot over medium-high heat, sauté onion and pumpkin or squash in olive oil until onion is soft, about 4 minutes. Add curry powder, cumin, chilies, and cloves and heat 1 minute, stirring frequently.

2. Reduce heat to medium and add water or vegetable broth and lentils. Cover and cook about 10–12 minutes, stirring occasionally.

3. Uncover and add tomatoes, green beans, and coconut milk, stirring well to combine. Heat uncovered 4–5 more minutes, just until tomatoes and beans are cooked.

4. Serve over rice or whole grains.

Black Bean Perfection

You can switch out the black beans for any other bean; try mixing it up with pinto beans, chickpeas, or Peruvian beans.

INGREDIENTS | SERVES 8

2 cups dried black beans

1 medium white onion, peeled and quartered

8 cloves garlic, peeled

Sodium Saver

Preparing beans from scratch drastically reduces your sodium intake in comparison to canned beans. One ½-cup serving of canned beans has approximately 350 milligrams sodium, compared to this recipe that has 0 milligrams added sodium. Be sure to keep this in mind if you are adding salt to your beans; each teaspoon of salt has approximately 2,300 milligrams sodium! If blood pressure is a concern of yours, try using lite salt or a salt substitute.

1. In a large pot filled with water, soak beans overnight.

2. Drain water, then refill the pot with fresh water and return beans to the pot.

3. Add onion and garlic cloves. Bring to a boil, then cover and simmer 2 hours. Serve beans with or without the onion and garlic.

4. If desired, purée drained beans, garlic, and onion in a food processor.

Kidney Bean and Chickpea Salad

*This marinated two-bean salad is perfect for summer picnics
or as a side for outdoor barbecues or potlucks.*

INGREDIENTS | SERVES 6

¼ cup olive oil

¼ cup red wine vinegar

½ teaspoon paprika

2 tablespoons lemon juice

1 (14-ounce) can chickpeas, drained and rinsed

1 (14-ounce) can kidney beans, drained and rinsed

½ cup sliced black olives

1 (8-ounce) can corn, drained and rinsed

½ medium red onion, peeled and chopped

1 tablespoon chopped fresh parsley

⅛ teaspoon salt

⅛ teaspoon ground black pepper

1. Whisk together olive oil, vinegar, paprika, and lemon juice.

2. In a large bowl, combine the chickpeas, beans, olives, corn, onion, and parsley. Pour the olive oil dressing over the bean mixture and toss well to combine.

3. Season with salt and pepper. Chill at least 1 hour before serving to allow flavors to mingle.

Cilantro Lime Rice and Bean Bowl

Layers of rice, beans, and veggies topped with all the fixings.
This dish is a quick and easy dinner you will surely enjoy.

INGREDIENTS | SERVES 4

1 cup uncooked rice

¼ cup cilantro, finely chopped

Juice of 1 medium lime

1 medium red onion, peeled and diced

1 medium serrano pepper, seeded and finely diced

1½ teaspoons olive oil

2 cups prepared black beans or canned black beans, drained and rinsed

1 cup corn, roasted

1 medium avocado, diced

1 medium Roma tomato, diced

¼ cup shredded Cheddar cheese (optional)

¼ cup green chili salsa (optional)

1. In a medium pot, prepare rice according to package instructions. Once fully cooked, add cilantro and lime juice and stir.

2. Meanwhile, in a medium skillet, sauté onion and pepper in olive oil over medium heat until lightly browned, about 7–8 minutes. Add black beans and corn, heating until warm, about 2–3 minutes.

3. Prepare rice bowl by layering rice, then bean mixture, and topping with avocado, tomato, cheese, and salsa if desired.

Skip the Rice

If you are feeling adventurous, try skipping the extra carbs, such as the rice in this recipe or bread on your sandwich. By cutting out the extras, you will save yourself 200–300 calories, and you'll also save your blood sugar from bouncing around due to the rapidly absorbed white carbs.

Black Bean Avocado Wrap

This wrap is also delicious when served warm. To heat, place tortilla with beans, quinoa, and feta cheese under the broiler for 1–2 minutes. Remove from broiler, add the remaining ingredients, and enjoy.

INGREDIENTS | SERVES 1

1 high-fiber tortilla

¼ cup prepared black beans or canned black beans, drained and rinsed

¼ cup cooked quinoa

1 tablespoon chopped cilantro

1 tablespoon diced red onion

2 tablespoons feta cheese

2 tablespoons diced tomatoes

¼ medium avocado, sliced

2 tablespoons green salsa (optional)

Place tortilla on a plate. Layer in all ingredients (including salsa, if desired) and roll up.

How to Pick That Tortilla

Unfortunately, most tortillas contain quite a bit of carbohydrates. Well, the good news is that with the recent health craze, manufacturers have come to the table with a few great low-carb tortillas. The great news for the blood sugar conscious is that the newer tortillas marketed to be low in carbs actually make tortillas more desirable. They are now lower in carbs and higher in fiber—a win-win for the blood sugar!

Super Fiber Wrap

This wrap is wonderful when served cold, so try preparing it the night before to take to work. You may want to add a drizzle of balsamic vinegar for extra flavor.

INGREDIENTS | SERVES 1

1 high-fiber tortilla

½ cup chopped spinach

2 teaspoons chopped sun-dried tomatoes

¼ cup canned chickpeas, drained and rinsed

1 tablespoon diced red onion

¼ cup chopped mushrooms

2 teaspoons shredded mozzarella cheese

2 teaspoons goat cheese crumbles

1. Heat tortilla in a medium skillet over medium heat.

2. Layer in the ingredients as listed, heating until all ingredients are warmed. Remove from heat and roll up.

CHAPTER 12

Main Dish Meals

Soy and Ginger Flank Steak

Soy and Ginger Flank Steak makes an excellent addition to any Asian-themed menu. Try mixing the sliced cooked steak into your next stir-fry just before serving.

INGREDIENTS | SERVES 4

1 pound lean London broil

1 tablespoon fresh ginger, minced

2 teaspoons fresh garlic, minced

1 tablespoon reduced-sodium soy sauce

3 tablespoons dry red wine

¼ teaspoon ground black pepper

½ tablespoon olive oil

Slicing Meats Against the Grain

Certain cuts of meat such as flank steak, brisket, and London broil have a distinct grain (or line) of fibers running through them. If you slice with the grain, the meat will seem tough and difficult to chew. These cuts of meat should always be thinly sliced across (or against) the grain so the fibers are cut through.

1. Marinate meat at least 3–4 hours in advance. Place meat, ginger, garlic, soy sauce, red wine, pepper, and olive oil in shallow baking dish. Coat meat with marinade on both sides.

2. Cover and refrigerate meat in marinade, turning meat once or twice during marinating so all marinade soaks into both sides of meat.

3. Lightly oil barbecue grill and preheat. Place flank steak on grill. Grill steak, turning once, until done to your preference. Medium-rare will take approximately 12–15 minutes. Slice meat diagonally and against grain into thin slices.

Pecan-Crusted Roast Pork Loin

Pork loin is a lean source of protein that fits perfectly into a balanced diet. Chopped walnuts or hazelnuts would make an excellent addition to this recipe if you don't have pecans on hand.

INGREDIENTS | SERVES 4

1 teaspoon olive oil

1 clove garlic, crushed

1 teaspoon brown sugar

¼ teaspoon dried thyme (optional)

¼ teaspoon dried sage (optional)

¼ teaspoon ground black pepper (optional)

¼ cup chopped or ground pecans

12 ounces boneless pork loin roast

Create a Celery Roasting Rack

If you prefer to bake a loin roast in a casserole alongside potatoes and carrots, elevate the roast on two or three stalks of celery. The celery will absorb any fat that drains from the meat so that it's not absorbed by the other vegetables. After cooking, discard the celery.

1. Put olive oil, crushed garlic, brown sugar, and optional seasonings (if using) in a heavy, freezer-style plastic bag. Work bag until ingredients are mixed. Add roast; turn in bag to coat. Marinate in refrigerator for several hours or overnight.

2. Preheat oven to 400°F.

3. Roll pork loin in chopped pecans; place in roasting pan. Make a tent of aluminum foil; arrange over pork loin, covering nuts completely so they won't char. Roast for 10 minutes, then lower heat to 350°F. Continue to roast for another 8–15 minutes, or until meat thermometer reads 150°F–170°F, depending on how well-done you prefer it.

Chicken Kalamata

Try serving this dish with large wedges of lemon to squeeze over the chicken. The bright acidic tang complements the Mediterranean flavors of this dish.

INGREDIENTS | SERVES 4

2 tablespoons olive oil

1 cup chopped white onion

1 teaspoon minced garlic

1½ cups chopped green peppers

1 pound boneless, skinless chicken breast, cut into 4 pieces

2 cups diced tomatoes

1 teaspoon oregano

½ cup chopped, pitted kalamata olives

1. Heat olive oil over medium heat in large skillet. Add onions, garlic, and peppers; sauté for about 5 minutes until onions are translucent.

2. Add chicken pieces; cook for about 5 minutes on each side until lightly brown.

3. Add tomatoes and oregano. Reduce heat and simmer 20 minutes.

4. Add olives; simmer an additional 10 minutes before serving.

Are Olives Counted As a Fruit or Vegetable?

The short answer is: neither! Even though olives are a fruit that grows on trees, their flesh is filled with a significant amount of oil and therefore is counted as a fat. Nine black olives or ten green olives equals one fat serving. The health benefits of olives (and olive oil) come from the monounsaturated fats they contain. Olives are usually cured in a brine, salt, or olive oil, so if you must watch your salt intake, be careful how many you eat.

Pesto Kale and Sweet Potatoes

This recipe is a complete meal all by itself. If you feel the need, add extra spinach or kale, or try serving this dish over a bed of fiber-rich grains, such as multicolored quinoa or brown rice.

INGREDIENTS | SERVES 8

1 medium white onion, peeled and sliced

¼ cup olive oil

4 medium sweet potatoes, sliced into ¼" pieces

4 bunches kale, stemmed and chopped

½ cup prepared pesto

¼ cup chopped walnuts

You Say Potato, I Say Pot-tat-to!

When compared to the ordinary white potato, the sweet potato is lower in calories and carbohydrates. The calories you save will keep your body on target for a healthy weight, and the lower carbohydrate content (and bonus fiber content) will keep your blood sugar stable and your metabolism functioning at its best. The sweet potato also provides a powerful punch of antioxidants that are associated with disease prevention.

1. In a large stockpot, sauté onion in olive oil over medium-low heat until softened, about 4 minutes.

2. Add sweet potatoes to pot, stirring well to coat with oil. Cover and cook 10–15 minutes until sweet potatoes are soft. Stir occasionally.

3. Add kale to the pot, mixing well. Cover and cook another 5 minutes or until kale has softened and wilted.

4. Remove from heat. Divide mixture into 8 bowls; top each bowl with 1 tablespoon pesto and ½ tablespoon walnuts.

Balsamic Dijon Orzo

Defying logic, this simple dish flavored with balsamic vinegar and Dijon mustard is somehow exponentially greater than the sum of its parts.

INGREDIENTS | SERVES 4

3 tablespoons balsamic vinegar

1½ tablespoons Dijon mustard

1½ tablespoons olive oil

1 teaspoon dried basil

1 teaspoon dried parsley

½ teaspoon dried oregano

1½ cups cooked orzo

2 medium tomatoes, chopped

½ cup sliced black olives

1 (15-ounce) can great northern or cannellini beans, drained and rinsed

½ teaspoon salt

¼ teaspoon ground black pepper

1. In a small bowl or container, whisk together vinegar, mustard, olive oil, basil, parsley, and oregano until well mixed.

2. Over low heat, combine orzo with balsamic dressing and add tomatoes, olives, and beans. Cook 3–4 minutes, stirring to combine.

3. Season with salt and pepper.

Oven-Roasted Spaghetti Squash with Veggies and Feta

Spaghetti squash may seem intimidating, but really the hardest part in preparing the spaghetti squash is cutting through the outer layer of the squash.

INGREDIENTS | SERVES 8

1 medium spaghetti squash

⅓ cup Smart Balance Buttery Spread

4 cups chopped spinach

4 medium Roma tomatoes, diced

2 medium green onions, sliced

1 medium red or green bell pepper, seeded and diced

¼ cup kalamata olives, chopped (optional)

½ cup feta cheese

1. Preheat oven to 400°F. Cut ends off spaghetti squash, then cut the squash in half lengthwise. Use a spoon to remove seeds. Place spaghetti squash face down in a glass casserole dish. Add ¼" water to dish and bake 40 minutes or until squash is easily pierced. You may flip right-side up and bake 10 minutes longer to enhance the flavor by gently browning some of the edges of the squash.

2. Allow squash to cool 10 minutes, until warm and able to be handled. Using a fork, gently comb out the spaghetti strands into a medium bowl. Add buttery spread to spaghetti, stirring well until buttery spread has melted.

3. Stir spinach into warm squash and allow spinach to wilt down. Add the remaining ingredients and stir.

Black Bean and Barley Taco Salad

Adding barley to this low-fat recipe gives it a bit of a whole-grain and fiber boost.

INGREDIENTS | SERVES 2

1 (15-ounce) can black beans, drained and rinsed

½ teaspoon cumin

½ teaspoon dried oregano

2 tablespoons lime juice

1 teaspoon hot chili sauce (optional)

1 cup cooked barley

1 head iceberg lettuce, shredded

¾ cup salsa

Handful tortilla chips, crumbled

2 tablespoons low-sugar Italian dressing (optional)

1. In a medium bowl, mash together beans, cumin, oregano, lime juice, and hot sauce until beans are mostly mashed, then combine with barley.

2. In a medium dish, layer lettuce with beans and barley mixture and top with salsa and tortilla chips. Drizzle with Italian dressing if desired.

Spicy Sweet Potato Tacos

This recipe is a meatless alternative to the usual beef tacos, which are higher in saturated fat. Give these potato tacos a try; you may be pleasantly surprised that you don't miss the meat!

INGREDIENTS | SERVES 4

4 medium sweet potatoes, cubed

2 tablespoons olive oil, divided

½ teaspoon salt

1 teaspoon garlic powder

1 medium white onion, peeled and chopped

1 medium serrano pepper, seeded and finely chopped

1 cup frozen roasted corn

1 (15-ounce) can black beans, drained and rinsed

8 corn tortillas

¼ cup feta cheese

1 medium tomato, diced

½ cup cilantro, chopped

Juice of 1 medium lime

1. Preheat oven to 400°F. Place sweet potatoes on a cookie sheet. Toss with 1 tablespoon olive oil, salt, and garlic powder and coat well. Bake 20 minutes or until lightly browned.

2. Meanwhile, in a medium saucepan, sauté onion and serrano pepper in remaining 1 tablespoon olive oil over medium heat 5 minutes or until lightly browned. Then add corn and black beans and cook 10 more minutes. Stir in sweet potatoes, cover, and lower heat to low for another 5 minutes.

3. Meanwhile, wrap corn tortillas in foil and place in oven 3–5 minutes to warm.

4. Assemble tacos by adding sweet potato filling and topping with feta cheese, tomato, cilantro, and lime juice.

Roasted Butternut Squash Pasta

For added flavor in this recipe, use roasted garlic instead of raw garlic.
Roasting garlic causes it to caramelize, adding a natural sweetness.

INGREDIENTS | SERVES 4

1 medium butternut squash
4 teaspoons extra-virgin olive oil
1 clove garlic, peeled and minced
1 cup chopped red onion
2 teaspoons red wine vinegar
¼ teaspoon dried oregano
2 cups cooked pasta (any kind)
Freshly ground black pepper (optional)

1. Preheat oven to 400°F. Cut squash in half and scoop out seeds. Using nonstick spray, coat 1 side of 2 pieces of heavy-duty foil large enough to wrap squash halves. Wrap squash in foil; place on a baking sheet. Bake 1 hour or until tender.

2. Scoop out baked squash flesh and discard rind; rough-chop. Add olive oil, garlic, and onion to a nonstick skillet. Sauté about 5 minutes until onion is transparent. (Alternatively, put oil, garlic, and onion in a covered microwave-safe dish; microwave on high 2–3 minutes.)

3. Remove skillet from heat; stir in vinegar and oregano. Add squash; stir to coat in onion mixture. Add pasta; toss to mix. Season with black pepper if desired.

Pesto Parmesan Quinoa

This dinner is so easy to prepare. It's a perfect choice for busy weeknights!

INGREDIENTS | SERVES 4

2 cups quinoa

4 cups vegetable broth

8 cups chopped spinach

2 medium Roma tomatoes, diced

⅓ cup prepared pesto

⅓ cup grated Parmesan cheese

1. In a medium pot, prepare quinoa with vegetable broth according to the package instructions.

2. Once quinoa is cooked, add spinach, stirring well, allowing the spinach to cook down.

3. Remove pot from heat and allow to cool 10 minutes. Mix in tomatoes, pesto, and cheese and serve warm.

Tuscan Pasta Fagioli

This traditional pasta and bean soup is an Italian classic. You could easily add shredded greens or chopped carrots and celery to boost the nutrition and fiber of this dish.

INGREDIENTS | SERVES 6

2 tablespoons olive oil

⅓ cup chopped white onion

3 cloves garlic, peeled and minced

½ pound medium tomatoes, chopped

5 cups low-sodium vegetable stock

¼ teaspoon freshly ground black pepper

3 cups canned cannellini beans, drained and rinsed

2½ cups whole-grain pasta shells

2 tablespoons grated Parmesan cheese

1. Heat olive oil in a large stockpot over medium heat; gently cook onion and garlic in oil until soft but not browned, about 4–6 minutes. Add tomatoes, vegetable stock, and pepper.

2. Purée 1½ cups cannellini beans in a food processor or blender; add to pot. Cover and simmer 20–30 minutes.

3. While stock is simmering, cook pasta until al dente; drain. Add remaining beans and pasta to stock; heat through. Serve with Parmesan cheese.

Broiled Tostadas with Avocado

If you have time, broil corn tortillas lightly rubbed with olive oil in place of the tostada rounds.

INGREDIENTS | SERVES 4

1 (15-ounce) can refried beans

8 small tostada rounds

¼ medium white onion, peeled and diced

1 medium jalapeño or serrano pepper, seeded and diced

¼ cup chopped fresh cilantro

1 medium Roma tomato, diced

¼ cup chopped Roasted Green Chilies (see recipe in Chapter 10, optional)

¼ cup crumbled queso blanco

1 medium avocado, diced

¼ cup tomatillo salsa (optional)

1. In a small saucepan, heat refried beans over medium heat until warmed through.

2. Preheat broiler.

3. Line a baking sheet with tostada rounds. Spread beans as bottom layer on rounds, then continue topping with remaining ingredients up to the queso blanco. Place under broiler 3–5 minutes until round is lightly browned and cheese is slightly melted. Top with avocado and salsa before serving.

Avocados Are Essential!

The avocado is a superfood that has received a bad reputation of being extremely high in fat. In actuality, it's the fat that makes the avocado so super! Fat is an essential component of your diet, whether you are on a lower-fat diet or a heart-healthy diet. The fat in avocado is mostly the good fats—essential, polyunsaturated, and monounsaturated, which have been found to lower the bad cholesterol and increase the good cholesterol. These are important for everyone, especially those with diabetes or who are at risk for heart disease.

Sweet Potato Enchiladas

Enchiladas freeze well, so make a double batch and thaw and reheat when you're hungry!

INGREDIENTS | SERVES 4

2 medium sweet potatoes, baked and diced

½ medium white onion, peeled and minced

3 cloves garlic, peeled and minced

1 (15-ounce) can black beans, drained and rinsed

2 teaspoons lime juice

2 tablespoons sliced green chilies (optional)

2 teaspoons chili powder

1 teaspoon cumin

1 (15-ounce) can green chili enchilada sauce

½ cup water

10–12 corn tortillas, warmed

Sweet Potato Burritos

Sweet potatoes and black beans make lovely vegan burritos as well as enchiladas. Omit the enchilada sauce and wrap the mixture in flour tortillas along with the usual burrito fixings.

1. Preheat oven to 350°F.

2. In a large bowl, combine sweet potatoes, onion, garlic, beans, lime juice, chilies, chili powder, and cumin until well mixed.

3. In a separate bowl, combine enchilada sauce and water. Add ¼ cup of this mixture to the sweet potato mixture and combine well.

4. Spread about ⅓ cup sauce in the bottom of a casserole or baking dish.

5. Place about ⅓ cup sweet potato mixture in each tortilla and wrap, then place in the casserole dish. Repeat until all filling is used.

6. Spread a generous layer of the remaining enchilada sauce over the top of the rolled tortillas, being sure to coat all the edges and corners well. You may have a little sauce leftover.

7. Bake 25–30 minutes. If enchiladas dry out while baking, top with more sauce.

Veggie-Loaded Sweet Potatoes

Mix it up! Add any other veggies into the mix, such as lightly steamed broccoli.
Top with walnuts if you have them in your pantry.

INGREDIENTS | SERVES 4

4 medium sweet potatoes

½ teaspoon salt, divided

½ medium red onion, peeled and chopped

1 tablespoon olive oil

4 cloves garlic, peeled and minced

4 cups chopped spinach

½ cup shredded Cheddar cheese

¼ cup plain, nonfat Greek yogurt

Seriously Sweet Potatoes

Most people think of sweet potatoes around Thanksgiving time, but really they should be a staple all year round. Sweet potatoes should be a vegetable/carb of choice, as they have a good amount of fiber, which helps slow down that mealtime blood sugar spike. But be sure to eat the skin, as that is where a lot of the fiber is hiding.

1. Preheat oven to 375°F. Rub potatoes with ¼ teaspoon salt, then wrap each potato in foil. Bake 50–60 minutes until easily pierced with a fork.

2. Meanwhile, in a medium skillet, sauté onion in olive oil over medium heat until caramelized, about 10 minutes.

3. Add garlic and remaining salt and sauté 30 seconds or until fragrant. Add spinach to pan, cover, and remove from heat.

4. Allow potatoes to cool 10–20 minutes. Remove foil and cut potatoes lengthwise. Fill potatoes with spinach mixture and top with cheese.

5. Return potatoes to oven 5–10 more minutes until cheese is golden brown. Top with a dollop of Greek yogurt.

Pesto Pizza

Lavash bread is so thin that it helps keeps your carb count low. Top your pizza with all your favorite vegetables. You can also throw in a few sun-dried tomatoes and pepperoncini for a zesty little kick.

INGREDIENTS | SERVES 4

1 sheet lavash bread
⅓ cup prepared pesto
½ cup chopped spinach
½ cup broccoli florets, steamed
2 medium Roma tomatoes, chopped
½ cup chopped artichoke hearts
8 kalamata olives, chopped
¼ cup feta cheese

1. Preheat oven to 400°F.

2. Place lavash bread on a cookie sheet. Spoon pesto on bread, then spread evenly using a spatula.

3. Top with spinach, broccoli, tomatoes, artichokes, olives, and feta.

4. Bake 10–12 minutes until edges of the bread are crispy.

Fruit or Vegetable?

The debate may go on whether the tasty tomato is a fruit or vegetable, but one thing is for sure: The tomato is a super food for your metabolism. Tomatoes are naturally low in calories and high in fiber, which is good for satisfying your appetite and maintaining a healthy weight. Tomatoes are also rich in antioxidants that fight free radicals.

Lemon Quinoa Veggie Salad

If you prefer to use fresh veggies, any kind will do. Steamed broccoli or fresh tomatoes would work well.

INGREDIENTS | SERVES 4

4 cups vegetable broth

1½ cups quinoa

1 cup frozen mixed vegetables, thawed

¼ cup lemon juice

¼ cup olive oil

1 teaspoon garlic powder

½ teaspoon sea salt

¼ teaspoon ground black pepper

2 tablespoons chopped fresh cilantro or parsley (optional)

1. In a large pot, bring vegetable broth to a boil. Add quinoa, cover, and simmer 15–20 minutes, stirring occasionally, until liquid is absorbed and quinoa is cooked. Add mixed vegetables and stir to combine.

2. Remove from heat and combine with remaining ingredients. Serve hot or cold.

Roasted Chickpea Pocket

*The sautéed onions and chickpeas can be refrigerated
until you are ready to prepare your pita. Serve hot or cold.*

INGREDIENTS | SERVES 4

½ medium red onion, peeled and diced

1 tablespoon olive oil

1 (15-ounce) can chickpeas, drained and rinsed

2 medium green onions, diced

½ teaspoon salt

1 teaspoon garlic powder

2 whole-wheat pitas, cut in half

4 cups chopped spinach

1 cup diced tomatoes

½ cup feta cheese

1. In a medium saucepan, sauté onion in olive oil over medium-high heat until lightly browned, about 5 minutes.

2. Add chickpeas and sauté 2–4 minutes, stirring frequently. Add green onions, salt, and garlic powder, stirring well and removing from heat.

3. Prepare pita pocket, filling with spinach, then bean mixture, and topping with tomatoes and feta cheese.

Spanish Artichoke and Zucchini Paella

Traditional Spanish paella is always cooked with saffron, but this version with zucchini, artichokes, and bell peppers uses turmeric instead for the same golden hue.

INGREDIENTS | SERVES 4

3 cloves garlic, peeled and minced

1 medium yellow onion, peeled and diced

2 tablespoons olive oil

1 cup uncooked white rice

1 (15-ounce) can diced or crushed tomatoes

1 medium green bell pepper, seeded and chopped

1 medium red or yellow bell pepper, seeded and chopped

½ cup chopped artichoke hearts

2 medium zucchini, sliced

2 cups vegetable broth

1 tablespoon paprika

½ teaspoon turmeric

¼ cup chopped parsley

½ teaspoon salt

1. In a large skillet, heat garlic and onion in olive oil 3–4 minutes until onion is almost soft. Add rice, stirring well to coat, and heat another minute, stirring to prevent burning.

2. Add tomatoes, bell peppers, artichokes, and zucchini, stirring to combine. Add vegetable broth and remaining ingredients, cover, and simmer 15–20 minutes until rice is done.

Beet and Avocado Roll-Up

This quick and easy beet salad is rolled up in a high-fiber tortilla for lunch on the go or dinner at home. Make an extra roll-up or two to have for another meal.

INGREDIENTS | SERVES 2

1 medium roasted beet, diced

2 cups chopped arugula or spinach

½ medium avocado, sliced

2 tablespoons goat cheese

1 tablespoon balsamic vinegar

2 tablespoons chopped walnuts

2 high-fiber tortillas

Divide ingredients evenly between two tortillas. Roll them up and enjoy.

Wild for Walnuts

Walnuts provide a good amount of omega-3 fatty acids and are rich in a variety of antioxidants. Walnuts may also help you keep your weight in balance because of the mix of fiber, protein, and fat, which will keep you feeling satisfied.

Sun-Dried Tomato Risotto with Spinach and Pine Nuts

The tomatoes carry the flavor in this easy risotto. But if you're a cook who keeps truffle, hazelnut, pine nut, or another gourmet oil on hand, now's the time to use it!

INGREDIENTS | SERVES 4

2 tablespoons olive oil

1 medium yellow onion, peeled and diced

4 cloves garlic, peeled and minced

1½ cups uncooked Arborio rice

5–6 cups vegetable broth

⅓ cup sun-dried tomatoes, sliced

½ cup chopped spinach

1 tablespoon chopped fresh basil (optional)

2 tablespoons Smart Balance Buttery Spread (optional)

2 tablespoons grated Parmesan cheese

⅛ teaspoon salt

⅛ teaspoon ground black pepper

¼ cup pine nuts

Sun-Dried Tomatoes

If you're using dehydrated tomatoes, rehydrate them first by covering in water for at least 10 minutes, and add the soaking water to the broth. If you're using tomatoes packed in oil, add 2 tablespoons of the oil to risotto at the end of cooking, instead of the Smart Balance Buttery Spread.

1. In a large skillet, heat olive oil over medium heat and add onion and garlic. Cook 2–3 minutes. Add rice and toast 1 minute, stirring constantly.

2. Add ¾ cup vegetable broth and stir to combine. When most of the liquid has been absorbed, add another ½ cup, stirring constantly. Continue adding broth ½ cup at a time until rice is cooked, about 20 minutes.

3. Add another ½ cup broth, tomatoes, spinach, and basil and reduce heat to low. Stir to combine well. Heat 3–4 minutes until tomatoes are soft and spinach is wilted.

4. Stir in spread and Parmesan cheese. Taste, then season lightly with a bit of salt and pepper.

5. Allow to cool slightly, then top with pine nuts. Risotto will thicken a bit as it cools.

Stuffed Green Chilies

If you like it spicy, go for the Anaheim or pasilla chili. If hot is not your style,
play it safe with the mild flavors of the green bell pepper.

INGREDIENTS | SERVES 4

½ medium white onion, peeled and diced

2 cloves garlic, peeled and minced

1 red bell pepper, seeded and diced

1 tablespoon olive oil

1 (15-ounce) can black-eyed peas, drained and rinsed

2 cups chopped spinach

½ cup roasted corn (optional)

4 medium Anaheim chilies or green bell peppers

¼ cup goat cheese crumbles

¼ cup diced black olives (optional)

¼ cup shredded Cheddar cheese

Easy on the Spice

You may notice the majority of the recipes in this book do not include too many extra spices. Challenge yourself to enjoy the flavors of your food without adding a whole lot of extra seasoning. This will help your taste buds wean off the overwhelming bold sweet and salty flavorings of processed foods.

1. Preheat oven 350°F.

2. In a medium skillet over medium heat, sauté onion, garlic, and red pepper in oil 7–10 minutes until soft. Add black-eyed peas, spinach, and corn and heat another 5 minutes. Remove from heat.

3. Cut the tops off the chilies; remove the inner webbing and seeds to form hollow cavities to stuff.

4. Mix goat cheese and olives with black-eyed pea mixture. Fill each chili with the black-eyed pea mixture, then top with cheese.

5. Place stuffed chilies in a casserole dish, upright if possible. Cover with foil and bake 20 minutes; uncover and bake another 10–15 minutes until chilies are tender.

Indian-Spiced Chickpeas with Spinach (Chana Masala)

This is a mild recipe, suitable for the whole family, but if you want to turn up the heat, toss in some minced fresh chilies or a hearty dash of cayenne pepper. It's enjoyable as is for a side dish or piled on top of rice or another grain for a main meal.

INGREDIENTS | SERVES 3

1 medium white onion, peeled and chopped

2 cloves garlic, peeled and minced

2 tablespoons Smart Balance Buttery Spread

¾ teaspoon coriander

1 teaspoon cumin

1 (15-ounce) can chickpeas, undrained

3 medium tomatoes, puréed, or ⅔ cup tomato paste

½ teaspoon curry powder

¼ teaspoon turmeric

¼ teaspoon salt

1 tablespoon lemon juice

1 bunch fresh spinach

1. In a large skillet, sauté onion and garlic in Smart Balance over medium heat until almost soft, about 2 minutes.

2. Reduce heat to medium-low and add coriander and cumin. Toast the spices, stirring, 1 minute.

3. Add chickpeas with liquid, tomatoes, curry powder, turmeric, and salt and bring to a slow simmer. Allow to cook until most of the liquid has been absorbed, about 10–12 minutes, stirring occasionally, then add lemon juice.

4. Add spinach and stir to combine. Cook just until spinach begins to wilt, about 1 minute. Serve immediately.

CHAPTER 13

Flavorful Fish

Sriracha-Seasoned Salmon

If you have a thicker cut of salmon, plan on cooking it a bit longer than instructed in this recipe. As a general rule, cooking time is 4–6 minutes per ½" thickness of salmon.

INGREDIENTS | SERVES 4

¼ cup Sriracha

¼ cup reduced-sodium soy sauce

2 cloves garlic, peeled and pressed (optional)

1 pound fresh salmon

½ cup diced pineapple (optional)

1. Mix together first 3 ingredients for marinade in a small bowl.

2. Pierce fish with a fork. Pour marinade over both sides of fish. Cover and refrigerate 30 minutes.

3. Preheat oven to 400°F.

4. Place fish on a foil-lined baking sheet. Bake 12–15 minutes until fish is easily flaked with a fork.

5. Top with pineapple if desired.

Do It for Your Heart

The general recommendation is to eat heart-healthy fish twice a week. Fish provides a good source of protein, the ever-so-popular omega-3 essential fatty acid, as well as a variety of vitamins and minerals. The omega-3 fat is extra special in the way it takes care of your heart, by lowering triglycerides and blood pressure as well as the risk of heart disease.

Pronto Pesto Fish and Foil

This is an all-in-one fish and veggie dinner, from start to finish in 20 minutes.

INGREDIENTS | SERVES 4

4 (4-ounce) salmon fillets

¼ cup prepared pesto

1 bunch asparagus, ends trimmed

4 cups chopped spinach

1 medium tomato, diced

1. Preheat oven to 400°F.

2. Lay out 4 pieces of foil. Place 1 salmon fillet in the middle of each piece of foil. Top each salmon fillet with 1 tablespoon pesto. Then top each fillet with 3–4 asparagus spears, 1 cup spinach, and ¼ tomato. Fold foil to seal all ingredients inside.

3. Bake 10–12 minutes until fish has lightened in color and is easily flaked with a fork.

White Wine Trout with Mushrooms

This flavorful trout is served with a white wine reduction and sautéed mushrooms over a bed of spinach. Top with a few red bell pepper slices for a presentation sure to delight.

INGREDIENTS | SERVES 4

1 pound trout

1 cup dry white wine

½ cup fresh parsley

1 cup chopped portabella mushrooms

1 tablespoon olive oil

½ teaspoon salt

½ teaspoon ground black pepper

4 cups chopped spinach

¼ medium red bell pepper, seeded and thinly sliced

Cooking with Wine

"I like to cook with wine. Sometimes I even put it in the food." If this funny saying rings true for you, then you probably already know what wine you like to cook with. For those who may need a little help, the most common dry white wines to cook with are Chardonnay, Pinot Grigio, and Sauvignon Blanc.

1. Preheat oven to 400°F. Place trout in a single layer in a baking dish. Cover fish with white wine and bake 15 minutes or until fish is cooked. Remove from oven. Pour the remaining white wine from the baking dish into a medium skillet.

2. Heat skillet over medium heat. Add parsley, mushrooms, olive oil, salt, and black pepper to white wine and simmer 10 minutes or until mushrooms are cooked.

3. Serve trout over a bed of spinach and top with white wine sauce and a few slices of red bell pepper.

Spicy "Fried" Fish Fillet

Many varieties of fish, including flounder, benefit from the distinctive flavor of lemon.
Serve slices of lemon to infuse flavor into this dish.

INGREDIENTS | SERVES 4

⅓ cup cornmeal

½ teaspoon salt

1 teaspoon chipotle seasoning

1 large egg

2 tablespoons 1% milk or milk substitute

1 pound flounder, cut into 4 pieces

2 tablespoons olive oil

1. Combine cornmeal, salt, and chipotle seasoning in a shallow dish.

2. Beat egg and milk together in a separate shallow dish.

3. Dip fish in egg mixture, then coat each fillet with cornmeal mixture.

4. Heat olive oil in a nonstick skillet over medium-high heat. Brown fillets until golden and crispy, about 6–7 minutes on each side.

Pineapple-Infused Shrimp Kabobs

Soaking the shrimp in pineapple juice and salt infuses it with a zesty flavor.

INGREDIENTS | SERVES 4

1 pound raw shrimp, deveined

1 cup pineapple juice

¼ teaspoon salt

1 cup cubed pineapple

2 medium carrots, peeled and chopped into 1" pieces

½ medium white onion, peeled and cut into 1" pieces

1 medium red bell pepper, seeded and cut into 1" pieces

1. In a small bowl, marinate shrimp in pineapple juice and salt 30 minutes–1 hour in the refrigerator.

2. Prepare kabobs, alternating marinated shrimp and remaining ingredients on skewers.

3. Lay shrimp skewers across heated grill. Close lid and cook 3–4 minutes, then turn. Remove skewers when shrimp have changed color and have cooked through.

It's a Dirty Job

Deveining shrimp is a dirty job, but some-one has got to do it! Take a knife and cut ¼" deep into the back of the shrimp, look-ing for the black or white vein. This isn't really a vein; it's actually the shrimp's GI tract, which contains waste. Using your fingers or a knife, remove the vein. Check the underside of the shrimp for the possible second vein and remove in the same way if present.

Blackened Salmon with Grilled Veggies

This recipe requires very little prep for a balanced grilled meal.

INGREDIENTS | SERVES 4

1 pound salmon, cut into 4 fillets

1 teaspoon blackened seasoning

1 cup broccoli florets

½ medium zucchini, sliced

1 medium red bell pepper, seeded and sliced into 1" pieces

1 cup sliced mushrooms

½ medium red onion, peeled and sliced

1 teaspoon olive oil

½ teaspoon salt

1 teaspoon garlic powder

1. Rub salmon with blackened seasoning and wrap in foil. In another piece of foil, place broccoli, zucchini, red pepper, mushrooms, and onion. Drizzle with olive oil, salt, and garlic powder, toss gently to evenly coat, and enclose in foil.

2. Place both foil wraps on a heated grill and cook 10–15 minutes until fish is cooked and vegetables are softened.

How Does Your Fish Rank?

There have been several rankings of the best fish, based on both the omega-3 content and the environment. Some of the best fish on the list are wild Alaskan salmon, rainbow trout, albacore tuna, and Pacific halibut. Of course, the environment is also susceptible to change, so vary the types of fish you choose.

Mahi-Mahi and Mango Street Tacos

Are you in a time crunch? Prepare the mango salsa and marinade ahead of time and store in the refrigerator until mealtime.

INGREDIENTS | SERVES 4

3 tablespoons olive oil

2 cloves garlic, peeled and minced

1 teaspoon cayenne pepper

½ teaspoon ground black pepper

½ teaspoon salt

2 medium limes, divided

¼ teaspoon lime zest

1 pound mahi-mahi

8 corn tortillas

½ cup shredded cabbage

½ cup chopped fresh cilantro

½ medium white onion, peeled and finely chopped

½ cup Mango Madness (see recipe in Chapter 14)

1. Mix together olive oil, garlic, cayenne, black pepper, salt, juice of 1 lime, and lime zest in a small bowl. Place fish in a single layer in a baking dish, pour marinade over fish, cover, and refrigerate 45–60 minutes.

2. Preheat oven to 375°F. Remove fish from marinade and place on a foiled-lined baking sheet and bake 10–12 minutes until fish flakes easily with a fork.

3. Fill each tortilla with fish, then top with remaining ingredients and remaining lime juice.

Hot Tortillas

Try heating the corn tortillas just before serving the tacos. Turn on broiler. Drizzle a pea-sized drop of olive oil on each corn tortilla, rub on both sides, and place under broiler. Heat tortillas 3–4 minutes, then flip. Remove after 5–6 minutes when tortillas are hot and somewhat crispy. You can also make your own corn tortilla chips the same way!

Barley Spinach Fish Bake

Brown rice would be a simple swap in this recipe if you do not have barley in your pantry. Alternatively, try serving with quinoa, millet, or farro.

INGREDIENTS | SERVES 4

½ tablespoon olive oil

¼ cup chopped green onion

1 clove garlic, peeled and minced

¼ teaspoon dried rosemary

¼ teaspoon dried marjoram

½ teaspoon salt, divided

1 cup cooked pearl barley

5 ounces frozen chopped spinach, thawed and drained

¼ cup sun-dried tomatoes, chopped

4 (12") squares aluminum foil

4 (4-ounce) cod fish fillets

3 tablespoons white wine

¼ teaspoon ground black pepper

Cooking Barley

Pearl barley takes longer to cook than quick-cooking barley, so you will want to prepare it in advance. To prepare: Bring ½ cup pearl barley and 1 cup water to a boil. Reduce heat, cover, and simmer 35–45 minutes until all water is absorbed. Pearl barley makes a good side dish on its own with the addition of spices or vegetables.

1. Preheat oven to 400°F (or a grill can be used).

2. Heat oil in a medium nonstick skillet; add green onion and sauté 2 minutes. Add garlic, rosemary, marjoram, and ¼ teaspoon salt; continue to cook another 3 minutes or until green onion is tender. Add cooked barley, spinach, and sun-dried tomatoes; mix well.

3. Place aluminum foil squares on work surface; place 1 fish fillet in the center of each square. Divide barley mixture equally; place on top of each fillet. Sprinkle with white wine, remaining salt, and pepper.

4. Fold aluminum foil loosely to enclose filling. Place packets on a baking sheet (or directly on grill if using a grill); bake 15 minutes or until fish is tender and flakes easily.

Wasabi-and-Ginger-Crusted Tilapia

The mild flavor of the tilapia goes perfectly with the bold flavors of wasabi and ginger.

INGREDIENTS | SERVES 4

2 teaspoons wasabi powder

1 tablespoon grated fresh ginger

2 tablespoons coconut flour

2 tablespoons Smart Balance Buttery Spread, melted

2 tablespoons water

¼ teaspoon salt

¼ teaspoon ground black pepper

1 pound tilapia fillets

4 cups chopped spinach

2 cups cooked rice

1 medium avocado, diced

1 teaspoon reduced-sodium soy sauce

1 teaspoon Sriracha

1. Preheat oven to 350°F.

2. In a small bowl, mix together the first 7 ingredients.

3. Lay tilapia fillets in a baking dish, then coat fish with wasabi mixture.

4. Bake 20–25 minutes until fish is cooked and easily flaked with a fork.

5. Serve fish over a bed of spinach and rice. Top with avocado, soy sauce, and Sriracha.

Crazy for Coconut

Coconut flour is an amazing blood sugar–conscious substitute for regular flour. It is high in fiber and low in total carbohydrates. It also adds a subtle but sweet coconut flavor to this dish.

Spicy Shrimp Wrap

Leftover coleslaw can be served as a side dish for another meal—double bonus!

INGREDIENTS | SERVES 4

1 teaspoon olive oil

½ medium white onion, diced

1 medium jalapeño or serrano pepper, seeded and minced

½ cup chopped fresh cilantro, divided

1 pound frozen cooked shrimp

1 (14-ounce) package coleslaw mix

1 cup roasted corn

½ cup diced green onion

1 cup diced tomatoes

½ cup ranch dressing

4 high-fiber tortillas

1 medium avocado, diced

2 tablespoons plain, nonfat Greek yogurt (optional)

1 medium lime

1. In a medium skillet over medium-high heat, heat oil and sauté onion, jalapeño, 2 tablespoons cilantro, and shrimp about 10 minutes or until shrimp is heated all the way through.

2. Meanwhile, in a medium bowl, mix together coleslaw mix, corn, green onion, tomatoes, and dressing.

3. If desired, heat tortillas under broiler 4–5 minutes until warm. Fill tortillas with shrimp, coleslaw mixture, avocado, Greek yogurt, and a squeeze of lime. Wrap up and enjoy.

Coleslaw Shortcut

If you feel up to it, you can always buy a head of red or green cabbage and a bag of carrots instead of the store-bought bagged coleslaw mix. You will definitely save money, but it may take just a bit more time.

Honey Dijon Tuna Salad

Substituting nonfat yogurt for mayonnaise cuts fat and calories considerably. With the addition of Dijon mustard, lemon juice, and honey, you won't even miss the mayonnaise!

INGREDIENTS | SERVES 1

¼ cup canned tuna in water, drained

½ cup diced celery

¼ cup diced white onion

¼ cup chopped red or green bell pepper

4 ounces plain, nonfat Greek yogurt

1 teaspoon Dijon mustard

1 teaspoon lemon juice

¼ teaspoon honey

1 tablespoon raisins (optional)

1 cup tightly packed chopped iceberg lettuce or other salad greens

1. Use a fork to flake tuna into a medium bowl. Add all other ingredients except lettuce; mix well. Serve over lettuce.

2. Alternate serving suggestion: Mix with ½ cup chilled cooked pasta before serving over lettuce.

Sweet-Potato-and-Walnut-Crusted Halibut

Pair this hearty fish with a light, leafy salad or side of something green.

INGREDIENTS | SERVES 4

1 medium baked sweet potato

1 cup chopped walnuts

¼ cup water

½ teaspoon salt

¼ teaspoon ground black pepper

1 tablespoon garlic powder

1 pound halibut

¼ cup prepared pesto (optional)

1. Place sweet potato, walnuts, water, salt, pepper, and garlic powder in a food processor and blend until smooth.

2. Preheat oven to 375°F. Coat halibut with sweet potato mixture and lay on a wire rack on top of a baking sheet. Bake 20–25 minutes until fish is cooked and outer coating is crispy. Serve topped with pesto if desired.

Grilled Salmon with Roasted Peppers

The wasabi marinade used in this recipe works well with chicken breasts and steak tips—meats that can withstand the pungent flavor of the horseradish.

INGREDIENTS | SERVES 4

4 (4-ounce) salmon steaks
Wasabi marinade (see sidebar)
2 large red bell peppers
1 tablespoon balsamic vinegar
½ teaspoon dried thyme
¼ teaspoon freshly ground black pepper

Wasabi Marinade

Wasabi, also known as Japanese horseradish, can be purchased in raw form or as a powder or paste. It adds a hot, pungent flavor to fish and works especially well with salmon. To make a marinade for salmon or other fish, mix 1 teaspoon wasabi powder (or paste) with 2 tablespoons low-sodium soy sauce, ½ teaspoon grated fresh ginger, and 1 teaspoon sesame oil. Coat fish with the marinade and grill.

1. Place salmon in a shallow dish. Mix together wasabi marinade; pour over salmon and cover both sides with marinade. Set aside.

2. Roast red bell peppers (see sidebar with Roasted Red Pepper Hummus recipe in Chapter 14). Once peppers are roasted and peeled, cut into strips and sprinkle with balsamic vinegar, thyme, and black pepper. Set aside.

3. Heat grill to medium. Remove salmon from the marinade and grill approximately 8 minutes on one side. Turn and grill on the other side until salmon is cooked and tender, about 4–5 minutes longer. Remove from heat.

4. Top each salmon steak with roasted red peppers.

Crab Cakes with Sesame Crust

These crab cakes make a stunning presentation.
Try serving over a bed of arugula with lemon wedges on the side.

INGREDIENTS | SERVES 5

1 pound lump crabmeat

1 large egg

1 tablespoon minced fresh ginger

1 small green onion, finely chopped

1 tablespoon dry sherry

1 tablespoon freshly squeezed lemon juice

6 tablespoons real or vegan mayonnaise

¼ teaspoon sea salt

¼ teaspoon freshly ground white pepper

1 teaspoon Old Bay Seasoning (optional)

¼ cup lightly toasted sesame seeds

1. Preheat oven to 375°F. In a large bowl, mix together crab, egg, ginger, green onion, sherry, lemon juice, mayonnaise, salt, pepper, and Old Bay Seasoning, if using.

2. Form mixture into 10 equal cakes. Spread sesame seeds over a sheet pan; dip both sides of cakes to coat them. Arrange cakes on separate baking sheet treated with nonstick spray. Typical baking time is 8–10 minutes, depending on thickness of cakes.

Simple Shrimp Salad

Purchasing frozen cooked shrimp will save you time and the hassle of deveining the shrimp.

INGREDIENTS | SERVES 4

1 teaspoon olive oil

1 pound frozen cooked shrimp

½ cup chopped fresh cilantro, divided

8 cups chopped spinach

½ cup diced red onion

½ cup diced tomatoes

¼ cup diced kalamata olives

¼ cup feta cheese

1 medium avocado, diced

¼ cup olive oil (optional)

¼ cup balsamic vinegar (optional)

1. In a medium skillet, heat 1 teaspoon olive oil and sauté shrimp and 2 tablespoons cilantro about 10 minutes or until shrimp is heated all the way through.

2. Meanwhile, in a medium bowl, combine remaining ingredients except ¼ cup olive oil and balsamic vinegar.

3. Portion salad into serving bowls and top with shrimp. If desired, dress with oil and vinegar.

Sun-Dried Tomato and Caper Fish Sauté

This dish pairs well with Extra Crispy Broccoli Florets (Chapter 10).

INGREDIENTS | SERVES 4

1 tablespoon olive oil

½ medium white onion, peeled and diced

1 pound tilapia, cut into 4 (4-ounce) fillets

4 cups chopped spinach

2 tablespoons diced sun-dried tomatoes

1 teaspoon capers

2 tablespoons goat cheese crumbles

1. Heat oil in a medium skillet over medium heat and sauté onion 10 minutes or until soft and lightly browned. Add tilapia fillets to pan, cook 4 minutes on one side, then flip fish over and cook another 4–5 minutes until fish is easily flaked with a fork.

2. Place 1 cup spinach on each plate, then top with fish, sun-dried tomatoes, capers, and goat cheese.

Careful with the Capers

Capers are little green flower buds that lend a salty punch to this dish. It is just important to keep a close eye on the amount used, as 1 tablespoon capers contains 240 milligrams sodium. That's quite a bit for such a little salty "pea."

Roasted Romaine and Mahi-Mahi

*Roasting romaine on the grill gives the fish a different look
and adds a delicious new taste to your usual salad.*

INGREDIENTS | SERVES 4

1 tablespoon olive oil

½ cup balsamic vinegar, divided

½ teaspoon salt, divided

½ teaspoon cracked black pepper, divided

8 small romaine hearts

1 pound mahi-mahi

¼ cup grated Parmesan cheese

1 cup diced tomatoes

¼ cup feta cheese

½ cup plain, nonfat Greek yogurt, seasoned with ranch dressing powder (optional)

1. In a small bowl, whisk together olive oil, ¼ cup balsamic vinegar, ¼ teaspoon salt, and ¼ teaspoon pepper. Brush romaine hearts with mixture.

2. Rub mahi-mahi with ¼ teaspoon each salt and pepper.

3. Place romaine hearts and fish on heated grill. Cook romaine hearts until lightly charred on the ends and fish until easily flaked with a fork, approximately 10 minutes.

4. Place two romaine hearts on each plate. Sprinkle with Parmesan cheese, tomatoes, and feta. Drizzle each serving with 1 tablespoon balsamic vinegar. Top with grilled mahi-mahi. Serve with additional balsamic vinegar or with ranch-flavored Greek yogurt if desired.

Salmon Fried Rice

*If you have leftover Sriracha-Seasoned Salmon (see recipe in this chapter),
you may use it in this recipe to transform it into a completely different meal.*

INGREDIENTS | SERVES 4

1 tablespoon olive oil

1 medium white onion, peeled and diced

2 cloves garlic, peeled and minced

½ pound cooked salmon, flaked into small pieces

½ cup frozen peas and carrots

¼ cup diced green onion

1 roasted green chili, diced (optional)

½ cup diced tomatoes

¼ cup chopped fresh cilantro

¼ cup roasted peanuts

1 teaspoon reduced-sodium soy sauce

1 teaspoon Sriracha

2 cups cooked brown rice

1. In a large skillet, heat olive oil over medium heat, sauté white onion 5 minutes, then add garlic, cooking an additional 2–3 minutes. Add salmon, peas and carrots, green onion, roasted chili, tomatoes, and cilantro, and heat 10 minutes.

2. Add peanuts, soy sauce, Sriracha, and brown rice, then remove from heat.

CHAPTER 14

Quick and Easy Appetizers

Roasted Red Pepper Hummus

Homemade roasted red peppers provide an amazing flavor for this quick and easy appetizer, but if you are in a time crunch, grab a jar of store-bought roasted red peppers. Serve with baked whole-grain pita chips or an assortment of veggies.

INGREDIENTS | SERVES 4

2 roasted red peppers or ½ cup jarred roasted red peppers

1 (15-ounce) can chickpeas, drained and rinsed

3 medium cloves garlic, peeled

2 tablespoons ground flaxseed

Juice of ½ medium lemon

1 teaspoon red pepper flakes

3 tablespoons olive oil

½ teaspoon sea salt

Combine all ingredients in a food processor and pulse until smooth and creamy.

Homemade Roasted Red Peppers

Roasting red peppers may seem like a challenge, but actually they really couldn't be easier. You get to burn them, so you really can't mess it up! Preheat broiler. Place whole peppers on a cookie sheet and broil for 20–30 minutes, turning 1–2 times, until skins are charred. Remove from heat, cool, then remove skins and seeds. You can keep them in the refrigerator for a few days or freeze them for later use.

Holy Guacamole

This recipe can be your everyday guacamole or your festive holiday guacamole with the added pop of color and sweetness from cranberries or pomegranate.

INGREDIENTS | SERVES 8–10

4 medium avocados

1 medium red onion, peeled and finely chopped

1 medium serrano pepper, finely chopped

3 medium Roma tomatoes, diced

½ cup chopped fresh cilantro

Juice of 1 medium lime

½ teaspoon salt

½ teaspoon ground black pepper

1 cup loosely packed dried cranberries or fresh pomegranate seeds (optional)

1. Mash avocados in a medium bowl. Add the next 7 ingredients, mixing well.

2. Add dried cranberries and refrigerate about 1 hour prior to serving.

Tomatillo Salsa

This salsa goes perfectly with guacamole, and is a great twist on traditional salsa recipes.

INGREDIENTS | SERVES 10

8 medium tomatillos, husks removed

1 medium serrano pepper, whole, stem removed

4 cloves garlic, peeled

½ cup chopped fresh cilantro

1 teaspoon sea salt

1 teaspoon garlic powder (optional)

Go for the Green!

Tomatillos are basically green tomatoes with a husk. Husks can be intimidating, but these are simple to handle. Just pull off the husk, rinse, and you are ready to go. No need to peel, chop, or seed tomatillos before cooking.

1. Place tomatillos, pepper, and garlic in a large stockpot and fill with water to cover. Bring to a boil over medium-high heat and cook 10–15 minutes until tomatillos are light green and soft.

2. Drain water from pot. Add ingredients from pot with the cilantro to a food processor and blend until a salsa-like consistency is acheieved.

3. Stir in salt and garlic powder if desired. Refrigerate until ready to serve.

Cucumber Slices with Smoked Salmon Cream

This is a simple yet elegant appetizer.
Fresh dill sprigs would make a flavorful and aromatic addition to this dish.

INGREDIENTS | MAKES ABOUT ½ CUP

2–3 medium cucumbers

1 ounce smoked salmon

8 ounces Neufchâtel cheese, at room temperature

½ tablespoon lemon juice

½ teaspoon freshly ground black pepper

1 teaspoon dried dill (optional)

1. Cut cucumbers into ¼" slices. Place on paper towels to drain while you prepare salmon cream.

2. Combine smoked salmon, Neufchâtel, lemon juice, and pepper in a food processor; blend until smooth.

3. Fit a pastry bag with tip; spoon salmon cream into the bag. Pipe 1 teaspoon salmon cream atop each cucumber slice. Garnish with dried dill if desired.

Mango Madness

Sweet mango paired with spicy salsa goes perfectly with fish, especially as a filling for fish tacos. It's also great with traditional tortilla chips!

INGREDIENTS | SERVES 8

1 large mango, peeled and diced

4 medium Roma tomatoes, diced

¼ cup finely chopped fresh cilantro

3 small avocados, diced

1 medium serrano pepper, seeded and finely chopped

¼ medium white onion, peeled and finely diced

Juice of ½ medium lemon

½ teaspoon sea salt

1 tablespoon garlic powder

1. Combine all ingredients and mix gently with a spoon.

2. Refrigerate 15–30 minutes prior to serving.

Onion Dip

This is a great dip for roasted green beans or carrots.

INGREDIENTS | SERVES 2

1 cup cottage cheese

2 tablespoons grated Parmesan cheese

1 tablespoon garlic powder

2 tablespoons dried onion flakes

1 teaspoon sea salt

½ teaspoon ground black pepper

1. Add all ingredients together in a medium bowl. Spoon into a food processor and pulse several times until cottage cheese is smooth.

2. Refrigerate at least 1 hour prior to serving.

Too Many Dairy Choices!

When it comes to shopping for dairy, you may find yourself in the grocery store feeling a little chilled and confused looking at all the different options available. Some are labeled 4% fat, full fat, reduced fat, 2% fat, light, skim, etc., but what does this all mean? Since dairy products come from an animal source, they are likely to contain saturated fat, unless the fat has been removed. Your goal is to keep your saturated fat intake low, so your best bet is to read the nutrition facts label and choose the option with the lowest saturated fat. This most likely will be the product labeled nonfat or skim.

Fruit Dip

Try this dip with an assortment of colorful fruits, especially strawberries, pineapple, pears, apples, peaches, grapes, and bananas. Top with chopped nuts, such as walnuts or pecans, for an added crunch.

INGREDIENTS | SERVES 6

1 cup plain, nonfat Greek yogurt

1 cup low-fat cream cheese

1 tablespoon honey

½ cup unsweetened applesauce or homemade cinnamon applesauce

2 tablespoons brown sugar

½ teaspoon cinnamon

1 tablespoon ground flaxseed

Combine all ingredients in a food processor and blend until smooth. Refrigerate 1 hour before serving.

Fried Zucchini Sticks

You don't have to deep-fry these zucchini sticks; just sauté them in a bit of oil if you prefer. This is a great appetizer or snack for kids!

INGREDIENTS | SERVES 4

½ cup all-purpose flour

¼ cup coconut flour

½ teaspoon garlic powder

¾ teaspoon Italian seasoning

¼ teaspoon salt

4 medium zucchini, cut into strips

¼ cup olive oil for frying

1. In a large bowl or pan, combine flours, garlic powder, Italian seasoning, and salt.

2. Lightly toss zucchini strips with the flour mixture, coating well.

3. Heat oil in a large skillet. When oil is hot, gently add zucchini strips to skillet.

4. Fry until lightly golden brown on all sides, 5–7 minutes.

Layered Greek Dip

This is a Greek spinoff of the traditional Mexican layered dip. Serve with whole-wheat pita bread, toasted whole-grain lavash, or zucchini slices.

INGREDIENTS | SERVES 8

½ medium white onion, peeled and diced

1 teaspoon olive oil

1 (15-ounce) can chickpeas, drained and rinsed

½ cup prepared hummus

½ medium cucumber, chopped

2 medium Roma tomatoes, diced

¼ medium red onion, peeled and diced

¼ cup pepperoncini peppers, sliced

¼ cup kalamata olives, sliced

¼ cup feta cheese crumbles

1. In a small skillet, sauté onion in olive oil over medium heat until caramelized, about 5 minutes. Add chickpeas, heating another 2–3 minutes.

2. Meanwhile, spread hummus evenly over the bottom of a circular serving dish. Top with sautéed onion and chickpeas.

3. Layer remaining ingredients and refrigerate before serving.

Three-Bean Dip

Serve this dip with homemade corn tortilla chips.
See sidebar with Mahi-Mahi and Mango Street Tacos in Chapter 13.

INGREDIENTS | SERVES 8

1 (15-ounce) can chickpeas, drained and rinsed

1 (15-ounce) can great northern beans, drained and rinsed

1 (15-ounce) can black beans, drained and rinsed

1 (15-ounce) can hominy, drained and rinsed

1 medium green bell pepper, seeded and diced

1 small red onion, peeled and diced

½ cup frozen roasted corn

2 medium Roma tomatoes, diced

1 medium serrano pepper, seeded and finely diced

½ cup Italian dressing

In a large bowl, combine all ingredients, tossing well to coat with Italian dressing. If desired, purée dip. Refrigerate at least 1 hour prior to serving.

More Serving Options

If you opt not to purée this dip, it can also serve as a topping for a taco, filling for a burrito, or a standalone spicy bean salad.

Balsamic Parsley Dip

This dip is amazing on whole-grain baguette or French bread, and it also makes a great topping for a salad or vegetables, especially mushrooms.

INGREDIENTS | SERVES 8

1 bunch parsley, finely chopped
1 bunch green onions, chopped
½ cup balsamic vinegar
½ cup olive oil
1 tablespoon garlic powder
½ teaspoon salt
¼ teaspoon cayenne pepper
½ teaspoon ground black pepper

Combine parsley and green onions in a large bowl. Add remaining ingredients, mixing well. Cover and refrigerate at least 1 hour prior to serving.

Tomato Basil Mini Skewers

This appetizer-style Caprese salad on a stick is both beautiful to look at and appealing to the taste buds.

INGREDIENTS | SERVES 8

1 pint cherry tomatoes
½ cup fresh basil leaves
1 cup cubed mozzarella
¼ cup balsamic vinegar
¼ cup olive oil
⅛ teaspoon salt
⅛ teaspoon ground black pepper

1. Alternate tomato, basil, and mozzarella on toothpicks.

2. Mix remaining ingredients to make balsamic dipping sauce.

Green and Black Olive Tapenade

Mediterranean olive tapenade can be used as a spread or dip for baguettes or crackers. If you don't have a food processor, you could also mash the ingredients together with a mortar and pestle or a large fork.

INGREDIENTS | MAKES 1 CUP

½ cup green olives

¾ cup black olives

2 cloves garlic, peeled

1 tablespoon capers (optional)

2 tablespoons lemon juice

2 tablespoons olive oil

¼ teaspoon dried oregano

¼ teaspoon ground black pepper

Process all ingredients in a food processor until almost smooth.

Spicy Black Bean Dip

Try this dip with a variety of chopped vegetable dippers.

INGREDIENTS | SERVES 8–10

2 cups puréed black beans or 1 (15-ounce) can refried black beans

¼ cup salsa

½ medium red onion, peeled and chopped

½ cup chopped fresh cilantro

1 cup diced tomatoes

1 medium jalapeño or serrano pepper, seeded and finely chopped

1 teaspoon lime juice

½ teaspoon salt

¼ teaspoon cayenne pepper

1 roasted green chili, diced (optional)

2 medium green onions, chopped (optional)

1 tablespoon plain, nonfat Greek yogurt (optional)

1. Mix together all ingredients except green chili, green onions, and Greek yogurt in a medium bowl.

2. Top with green chili, green onion, and a dollop of Greek yogurt if desired.

Sweet and Savory Rosemary Cashews

These sweet and savory cashews provide a nice alternative to the traditional chip-and-dip appetizers.

INGREDIENTS | MAKES 4 CUPS

1 pound raw cashews

2 tablespoons Smart Balance Buttery Spread, melted

¼ cup minced fresh rosemary

2 tablespoons brown sugar

1 teaspoon cayenne pepper

1 teaspoon salt

Why Smart Balance?

You may notice the reoccurring ingredient of Smart Balance Buttery Spread throughout this book, but why is this product the preferred butter choice? If you read the ingredient list of this product, you will see why. It is a nice blend of canola, palm, flax, fish, soy, and olive oils, providing a good balance of fat, including an excellent source of omega-3 fatty acids. And they were able to sneak some vitamin D in there for an added bonus.

1. Preheat oven to 375°F. Line a baking sheet with cashews and roast in oven 15 minutes or until golden brown.

2. Meanwhile, mix together remaining ingredients in a medium bowl. Once cashews are ready, add to the bowl with rosemary mixture and toss gently to coat. Allow to cool before serving or storing in an airtight container with a lid. Eat within a few days.

Black-Eyed Pea Dip

This fiber-rich black-eyed pea salsa can help balance your blood sugar level.
Serve this dip with baked tortilla chips or as a standalone side dish.

INGREDIENTS | MAKES 4 CUPS

2 tablespoons olive oil

1 medium white onion, peeled and diced

1 medium jalapeño or serrano pepper, seeded and diced

1 cup roasted corn

2 cups prepared black-eyed peas or 1 (15-ounce) can black-eyed peas, drained and rinsed

¼ cup chopped fresh cilantro

1 cup diced tomatoes

1 medium avocado, diced

Juice of 1 medium lime

¼ teaspoon red pepper flakes

½ teaspoon salt

1 teaspoon garlic powder

1. Heat oil in a medium skillet over medium-low heat; add onion and jalapeño and sauté 15–20 minutes until onion has caramelized, adding a little more oil as needed.

2. Add corn and black-eyed peas to skillet; cook 5–10 minutes, then remove from heat and allow to cool.

3. In a medium bowl, mix cooled black-eyed pea mixture with cilantro, tomatoes, and avocado. Season with remaining ingredients, mixing well. Chill in the refrigerator before serving.

Crispy Sweet Onion Lavash

This decadent lavash flatbread appetizer is so simple to make.
This could also be a quick weeknight dinner served with some vegetables.

INGREDIENTS | SERVES 8

2 tablespoons olive oil, divided

1 medium sweet onion, sliced into thin crescents

1 cup diced mushrooms

1 slice lavash bread

½ cup chopped fresh parsley

¼ cup goat cheese

1. In a medium skillet, heat 1 tablespoon olive oil over medium-low heat. Sauté onion 15 minutes, then add mushrooms; sauté another 5–7 minutes.

2. Preheat oven to 400°F. Lay lavash bread on a baking sheet, then top with remaining 1 tablespoon olive oil, spreading evenly over bread. Top with drained onion and mushroom mixture, parsley, and goat cheese. Bake 10 minutes, then cut and serve.

Artichoke Dip

*For a variation on this recipe, you can use ¼ cup
roasted red peppers instead of sun-dried tomatoes.*

INGREDIENTS | MAKES ABOUT 1 CUP

1 cup artichoke hearts, drained

1 tablespoon chopped red onion

1 tablespoon chopped sun-dried
tomatoes

1 tablespoon real or vegan mayonnaise

1 tablespoon reduced-fat sour cream

2 teaspoons grated Parmesan cheese

1 teaspoon lemon juice

½ teaspoon minced garlic

1 tablespoon olive oil

Put all ingredients in food processor; blend until smooth.
Chill before serving.

CHAPTER 15

Sinless Sweets

Sautéed Apples and Pears

On a busy night, this dessert treat can be sweetly sizzled up in minutes—without the guilt. This dish has a healthy balance of fruit and nuts, without the added fat and carbs that usually come with apple pie or cobbler.

INGREDIENTS | SERVES 6

2 apples, thinly sliced

2 pears, thinly sliced

1½ tablespoons Smart Balance Buttery Spread

¼ cup chopped walnuts

1 teaspoon cinnamon

1. In a medium skillet over medium heat, sauté apples and pears in buttery spread until soft and lightly browned, approximately 5–10 minutes.

2. Add walnuts to the pan and season mixture with cinnamon. Sauté 1 additional minute.

Don't Forget the Cinnamon

Usually the foods that maximize your metabolism are colorful foods loaded with amazing health properties, but don't let the finely ground, brown cinnamon powder fool you. Just ¼–1 teaspoon cinnamon a day can drastically improve your glucose metabolism, meaning it helps the body use insulin efficiently, taking the glucose out of the blood and into the cells for energy. By eating cinnamon daily, you can keep your blood sugar at a more stable level, reducing your risk for diabetes. As an added bonus, cinnamon also has been found to reduce the fat in your blood, including cholesterol and triglycerides.

Dessert Dates with Almond Butter

If you want to add extra fiber and protein with chia seeds, you may need to add a little additional water or almond milk to get the purée to your desired consistency.

INGREDIENTS | SERVES 4

8 dates, pitted

¼ cup almond butter

1 teaspoon unsweetened cocoa powder

1 tablespoon shelled hemp seeds, ground flaxseed, and/or chia seeds (optional)

2 tablespoons almond milk

1 teaspoon cinnamon

4 small cinnamon sticks (optional)

Almond Butter Addiction

If you haven't tried almond butter yet, then you are in for a treat. Natural almond butter may be a bit of an acquired taste if you are used to the usual processed peanut butter that has extra additives. Just one word of caution: Brace yourself for the price, but it is worth it—your heart and body will agree!

1. Mix together all ingredients except cinnamon sticks in food processer and blend.

2. Serve a small dollop in a dessert dish with a cinnamon stick.

Easy Banana Date Cookies

The daily fast during Ramadan is traditionally broken with a date at sunset, and a version of these simple, refined sugar–free cookies is popular in Islamic communities in northern Africa, though almonds are traditionally added.

INGREDIENTS | MAKES 1 DOZEN COOKIES

1 cup chopped pitted dates

1 medium banana

¼ teaspoon vanilla extract

1¾ cups coconut flakes

1. Preheat oven to 375°F. Cover dates in water and soak 10 minutes or until softened. Drain.

2. Combine dates, banana, and vanilla in a food processor and blend until almost smooth. Stir in coconut flakes by hand until thick. You may need a little more or less than 1¾ cups.

3. Drop by generous tablespoonfuls onto a cookie sheet. Bake 10–12 minutes or until lightly brown. Cookies will be soft and chewy.

No-Bake Peanut Butter Flax Balls

This recipe sneaks a few healthy ingredients into this after-dinner sweet treat.

INGREDIENTS | SERVES 4

¼ cup ground flaxseed

¼ cup raisins

¼ cup grated carrots

¼ cup quick-cooking steel cut oats

2 tablespoons chia seeds

2 tablespoons honey

¼ cup peanut butter

In a medium bowl, mix together all ingredients. Roll dough into ½" balls and place on sheet pans. Refrigerate 4–8 hours prior to serving.

High-Five for Flax!

Flaxseed is a lower-carbohydrate grain, packed with protein, fiber, and essential fats. Researchers have found that adding flaxseed to your diet is linked to lowering your blood cholesterol as much as a medication! With heart disease topping the list of causes of death, it seems that adding a little ground flaxseed to your meal may be a good idea. Flaxseed is also rich in fiber, which has been found to benefit your blood sugar as well. Intake of flaxseed daily reduces hemoglobin A1c levels, which lowers your risk of type 2 diabetes.

Homemade Cinnamon Applesauce Dessert

This applesauce can be served plain or as a dessert with the extra fixings.
If cocoa is not your favorite, trying mixing in sliced strawberries instead.

INGREDIENTS | SERVES 4

6 medium apples, cored and quartered

1 cinnamon stick

4 tablespoons shelled hemp seeds

4 teaspoons unsweetened cocoa powder

4 teaspoons ground flaxseed

1 teaspoon honey

Why Not Just Buy from the Store?

Making applesauce at home has its advantages over the store-bought versions. Probably the most important one is the sugar advantage. Store-bought applesauce may add sugar or high fructose corn syrup, and when you are making yours at home you can obviously leave these out. Be sure to stock up on apples when they are on sale to make this a cost-efficient advantage as well. Store applesauce in the refrigerator and use within 7–10 days.

1. To make applesauce, add apples and cinnamon stick to a large stockpot filled with water. Bring to a boil, then cover and reduce heat. Simmer 30–40 minutes until apples are softened.

2. Allow apples to cool. Discard cinnamon stick. Once cooled, strain apples and purée in food processor.

3. To serve, fill each bowl with 1 cup applesauce and top with 1 tablespoon hemp seeds, 1 teaspoon cocoa powder, and 1 teaspoon flaxseed. Drizzle with honey.

Coconut Chia Pudding

Double, triple, or quadruple this recipe—whatever you need to serve this fiber- and essential fatty acid–rich coconut treat to everyone at your table.

INGREDIENTS | SERVES 1

2 tablespoons chia seeds

1 cup unsweetened coconut milk

2 teaspoons unsweetened cocoa powder

1 tablespoon ground flaxseed

1 tablespoon coconut flakes

¼ teaspoon honey

Mix together all ingredients. Cover, shake well, and refrigerate 12–24 hours until pudding consistency is reached.

Key Lime Pie

This is a sweet lime treat with some serious substitutions to reduce the calorie intake of the usually high-calorie dessert.

INGREDIENTS | SERVES 10

1 cup graham cracker crumbs

1 tablespoon plus ½ cup Splenda Granulated, divided

2 tablespoons Smart Balance Buttery Spread, melted

½ teaspoon lime zest

6 ounces low-fat cream cheese

1 package sugar-free instant vanilla pudding mix

½ cup unsweetened coconut milk

1 cup key lime juice (5–6 limes), divided

1 tablespoon Knox Unflavored Gelatine

1. Preheat oven to 350°F.

2. Prepare graham cracker crust: In a large bowl, combine graham cracker crumbs and 1 tablespoon Splenda. Add melted Smart Balance; mix well. Press crumbs into 9" pie plate with the help of a flat surface such as the bottom of a glass. Bake 10 minutes; remove from oven and cool.

3. In a food processor, combine lime zest and ½ cup Splenda. Add cream cheese; process for 30 seconds. Add pudding mix and coconut milk; blend well.

4. Pour ¼ cup lime juice into a small measuring cup or bowl; heat in microwave for 1 minute. Add gelatine to heated juice; dissolve completely.

5. Mix dissolved gelatine in remaining lime juice. Turn on food processor; pour lime juice into mixture slowly. Process until all ingredients are well combined.

6. Pour filling into pie shell; refrigerate 3–4 hours before serving. If desired, top with light whipped cream.

Cinnamon Sweet Almonds

Oven-roasted almonds seasoned to sweet perfection.
Enjoy a few almonds to curb your sweet tooth.

INGREDIENTS | SERVES 16

2 tablespoons Smart Balance Buttery Spread, melted

1 teaspoon honey

1 teaspoon unsweetened coconut milk

4 cups raw almonds

1 tablespoon cinnamon

1 tablespoon shelled hemp seeds

2 tablespoons ground flaxseed

1. Preheat oven to 300°F.

2. Mix buttery spread, honey, and coconut milk in a medium bowl.

3. Meanwhile, line a baking sheet with foil. Spread almonds on the sheet, then coat evenly with coconut milk mixture. Sprinkle with cinnamon, hemp seeds, and flaxseed and toss to evenly coat.

4. Roast 15–20 minutes. Allow to cool before serving or storing.

Apple Cookies with a Kick

These apple cookies are packed with spice. Serve them warm on chilly fall or winter days.

INGREDIENTS | MAKES 24 COOKIES

1 tablespoon ground flaxseed

¼ cup water

¼ cup firmly packed brown sugar

⅛ cup granulated sugar

¾ cup canned pinto beans, drained

⅓ cup unsweetened applesauce

2 teaspoons baking powder

⅛ teaspoon sea salt

1 teaspoon cinnamon

½ teaspoon nutmeg

¼ teaspoon ground cloves

¼ teaspoon ground allspice

1 cup coconut flour

1 medium Golden Delicious apple, peeled and chopped

1 cup dried sunflower seed kernels (unroasted, unsalted)

Creative Substitutions

Adding nuts and, of all things, beans to dessert recipes increases the amount of protein and fiber. Just because it's dessert doesn't mean it has to be all empty calories.

1. Preheat oven to 350°F.

2. Put flaxseed and water in a microwave-safe container; microwave on high 15 seconds or until mixture thickens and has the consistency of egg whites. Add flaxseed mixture, sugars, beans, and applesauce to a medium mixing bowl; mix well.

3. Sift together dry ingredients; fold into bean mixture. (Do not overmix; this will cause cookies to become tough.)

4. Fold apple and sunflower seeds into batter.

5. Drop batter by teaspoonfuls onto a baking sheet treated with nonstick spray; bake 12–18 minutes.

Berry Cheesecake Parfait

If berries are not in season, try making this parfait with thawed, frozen berries.

INGREDIENTS | SERVES 4

1 package sugar-free cheesecake pudding, prepared

2 cups mixed berries

1 medium banana

1 cup fat-free whipped topping

½ cup high-fiber cereal

2 teaspoons unsweetened cocoa (optional)

1. Portion pudding into 4 parfait cups. Top each serving with ½ cup berries and ¼ sliced banana.

2. Top each parfait with ¼ cup whipped topping, 2 tablespoons cereal, and ½ teaspoon cocoa if desired.

Let Fiber Be Your Guide

Quaker Corn Bran or other high-fiber cereal gives this parfait a crunchy touch. If the cereal aisle seems overwhelming, just start reading the boxes to see if you can find the cereal with >3 grams fiber per serving.

Cocoa-Nut-Coconut No-Bake Cookies

Have the kids help you shape these into little balls, and try not to eat them all along the way!

INGREDIENTS | MAKES 2 DOZEN COOKIES

¼ cup Smart Balance Buttery Spread

½ cup almond milk

1 cup granulated sugar

1 cup Splenda

⅓ cup unsweetened cocoa powder

½ cup peanut butter (or other nut butter)

½ teaspoon vanilla extract

3 cups quick-cooking oats

½ cup finely chopped walnuts or cashews

½ cup coconut flakes

1. Line a baking sheet with wax paper.

2. In a medium saucepan over medium heat, melt buttery spread with almond milk and add sugar, Splenda, and cocoa powder. Bring to a quick boil to dissolve sugar, then reduce heat to low and stir in peanut butter just until melted.

3. Remove from heat and stir in remaining ingredients. Allow to cool slightly.

4. Spoon about 3 tablespoons of mixture at a time onto wax paper and press lightly to form a cookie shape. Chill until firm.

Minty Fruit Frenzy

This fruit salad features a rainbow of color and a minty twist.

INGREDIENTS | SERVES 8

2 cups sliced strawberries

2 medium mangos, peeled and diced

1 cup blueberries

2 medium kiwis, peeled and diced

1 cup sliced grapes

2 cups diced watermelon

2 cups diced cantaloupe

2 tablespoons finely chopped fresh mint

In a medium bowl, combine all ingredients and refrigerate until ready to serve.

Triple C Lover

Chocolate chip cookies with an added C for coconut! This is really two recipes in one. You can do a cookie switch-a-roo by using white chocolate chips and macadamia nuts instead.

INGREDIENTS | MAKES 3 DOZEN COOKIES

1 cup Crisco Butter Flavor
¾ cup granulated sugar
¾ cup brown sugar
2 large eggs
1 teaspoon vanilla extract
1 cup coconut flour
1 cup whole-wheat flour
¼ cup ground flaxseed
1 teaspoon baking soda
1 teaspoon salt
1 cup semi-sweet chocolate chips
½ cup chopped walnuts

"But I Only Had One!"

You may not feel too guilty if you eat just one cookie. But what if that cookie is the size of three cookies, giving you an extra 400–500 calories? When it comes to dessert, especially cookies, be sure to keep a close eye on the portion size. A cookie should be small, about the size of a half dollar. If you have a sweet tooth, trying baking up just one batch of cookies and freezing the leftover dough for later. This way, you avoid the cookie jar sabotage!

1. Preheat oven to 375°F.

2. In a medium bowl, mix together the first 5 ingredients by hand or with a mixer until creamy.

3. In a separate bowl, mix together both flours, flaxseed, baking soda, and salt.

4. Add the dry ingredients to the creamy mixture in a few batches until all ingredients are mixed together.

5. Fold in chocolate chips and walnuts.

6. Scoop dough by the teaspoon onto a baking sheet. Bake 12–16 cookies per batch, leaving space between each cookie. Bake 8–10 minutes until lightly browned. Allow to cool a few minutes on baking sheet, then move to a wire rack.

Popcorn and a Movie

This is a sweet and salty—and not to mention, high-fiber—popcorn treat.

INGREDIENTS | SERVES 4–6

2 tablespoons olive oil

⅔ cup popcorn kernels

1 tablespoon unsweetened cocoa powder

2 teaspoons honey

½ teaspoon salt

Just Say No to the Mystery Bag!

Microwave popcorn has been found to contain carcinogens in the butter flavoring and in the popcorn bag that are sneaking into the popcorn. It is a much better health option to make homemade popcorn to avoid these cancer risks. You will find that homemade popcorn is simple to pop up, and better yet, you know exactly what is and is not in it!

1. Heat olive oil and 4 popcorn kernels in a heavy pot with a lid over medium-high heat. Once 4 kernels pop, remove them from pot and add ⅔ cup popcorn kernels. Shake pot to evenly distribute kernels, then continue to shake every minute or so. Once popping slows down to every 3 seconds, remove from heat.

2. Pour popcorn into a bowl and season with remaining ingredients.

Chocolate-Dipped Delight

Substitute pineapple, pears, bananas, berries, oranges, or grapes for the strawberries for some variety. You may also want to dip a few nuts while you are at it!

INGREDIENTS | SERVES 4

½ cup dark chocolate chips

1 tablespoon Smart Balance Buttery Spread

1 teaspoon water (optional)

1 pint strawberries

¼ cup ground flaxseed

¼ cup coconut flakes or chopped walnuts (optional)

1. Heat chocolate chips and buttery spread in a medium saucepan over low heat, stirring constantly. Add water if mixture becomes too thick. Once melted, begin dipping strawberries in chocolate, then dip in flaxseed and coconut or walnuts if desired.

2. Place on waxed paper to allow chocolate to harden.

APPENDIX A

Sample Blood Sugar Meal Plans

Sunday

Breakfast: Breakfast Salad (Chapter 6)

Morning Snack: 1 cup carrots, 1 ounce almonds (22 almonds)

Lunch: Black Bean Avocado Wrap (Chapter 11), cucumber slices with a squeeze of lime juice

Afternoon Snack: Chia-C Water (Chapter 7), 1 cup frozen grapes

Dinner: Pesto Kale and Sweet Potatoes (Chapter 12), Sautéed Apples and Pears (Chapter 15)

Monday

Breakfast: Baked Apple Cinnamon Oatmeal Muffins (Chapter 6), 1 cup strawberries

Morning Snack: Mango Smoothie (Chapter 7)

Lunch: Pesto Kale and Sweet Potatoes (Chapter 12)

Afternoon Snack: Give Me a Beet (Chapter 8)

Dinner: Sweet and Spicy Baked Potato Coins (Chapter 10), Rainbow Salad with Cashews (Chapter 8)

Tuesday

Breakfast: Berry Nutty Smoothie (Chapter 7)

Morning Snack: Give Me a Beet (Chapter 8)

Lunch: Double Roasted Corn and Chickpea Salad (Chapter 8)

Afternoon Snack: Sweet and Spicy Baked Potato Coins (Chapter 10)

Dinner: Extra Crispy Broccoli Florets (Chapter 10), Super Fiber Wrap (Chapter 11)

Wednesday

Breakfast: Honey Butter Banana (Chapter 6)

Morning Snack: Roasted Red Pepper Hummus (Chapter 14), 1 cup cucumber slices

Lunch: Super Fiber Wrap (Chapter 11), ½ cup red pepper slices

Afternoon Snack: Watermelon Basil Salad (Chapter 8)

Dinner: Curried Kale and Lentil Stew (Chapter 9), Quick-Roasted Carrots (Chapter 10), Cinnamon Sweet Almonds (Chapter 15)

Thursday

Breakfast: Baked Apple Cinnamon Oatmeal Muffins (Chapter 6), 1 cup cubed watermelon with blueberries

Morning Snack: Sweet Green Smoothie (Chapter 7)

Lunch: Simple Shrimp Salad (Chapter 13), 1 cup strawberries

Afternoon Snack: Quick-Roasted Carrots (Chapter 10)

Dinner: Mahi-Mahi and Mango Street Tacos (Chapter 13), Holy Guacamole (Chapter 14), Balsamic Brussels (Chapter 10)

Friday

Breakfast: Avocado Toast (Chapter 6)

Morning Snack: Watermelon Basil Salad (Chapter 8)

Lunch: Curried Kale and Lentil Stew (Chapter 9), ½ cup red pepper slices

Afternoon Snack: Holy Guacamole (Chapter 14), 1 cup cauliflower florets

Dinner: Vegetable Curry (Chapter 10)

Saturday

Breakfast: Triple B–Breakfast Bean Bowl (Chapter 6)

Morning Snack: For the Love of Cucumber (Chapter 8)

Lunch: Rainbow Salad with Cashews (Chapter 8)

Afternoon Snack: 1 medium apple, sliced, 1 tablespoon almond butter, 1 teaspoon flaxseed, ¼ teaspoon cinnamon, drizzle of honey

Dinner: Sriracha-Seasoned Salmon (Chapter 13), Zesty Chili Corn on the Cob (Chapter 10), Spinach-Stuffed Mushrooms (Chapter 10)

High-Fiber and High-Protein Foods

Food	Serving Size (Cooked)	Fiber (Grams)	Protein (Grams)
Black beans	1 cup	15	15
Kidney beans	1 cup	11	15
Lima beans	1 cup	9	12
Chickpeas	1 cup	13	15
Black-eyed peas	1 cup	8	5
Edamame	1 cup	8	17
Pinto beans	1 cup	15	15
Lentils	1 cup	16	18
Green peas	1 cup	5	5
Almonds	1 ounce	4	6
Pistachio nuts	1 ounce	3	6
Cashews	1 ounce	1	4
Peanuts	1 ounce	2	7
Walnuts	1 ounce	2	7
Brazil nuts	1 ounce	2	4
Sunflower seeds	1 ounce	3	6
Pumpkin seeds	1 ounce	5	5
Sesame seeds	1 tablespoon	1	2
Flaxseed	1 tablespoon	2	1
Almond butter	1 tablespoon	2	3
Peanut butter	1 tablespoon	1	3
Sunflower seed butter	1 tablespoon	1	3
Hummus	1 tablespoon	1	1

Seasonal Produce Grocery List

SEPTEMBER TO NOVEMBER		
Fruit	**Serving Size**	**Fiber (Grams)**
Cherries	10 each	1.6
Cranberries	1 cup	4
Grapes	1 cup	0.9
Pears	1 medium	4
Pineapple	1 cup	1.9
Pomegranate	1 medium	0.9
Pumpkin*	½ cup	1.3
Vegetables	**Serving Size**	**Fiber (Grams)**
Broccoli	½ cup	1.3
Brussels sprouts*	½ cup	2
Cauliflower	½ cup	1.3
Lettuce	½ cup	0.5
Mushrooms	½ cup	0.4
Squash*	½ cup	1.3
Sweet potatoes	1 medium	3.4
Swiss chard	½ cup	1.8
Turnips	½ cup	1.6

(*means cooked)

DECEMBER TO FEBRUARY		
Fruit	**Serving Size**	**Fiber (Grams)**
Dates	10 each	6.2
Grapefruit	½ medium	1.4
Kiwi	1 medium	2.6
Mandarin oranges	2 small	2.8
Pear	1 medium	4
Tangerine	1 medium	1.9
Vegetables	**Serving Size**	**Fiber (Grams)**
Brussels sprouts*	½ cup	2
Collard greens*	1 cup	3.6
Kale*	½ cup	1.3
Leeks	¼ cup	0.5
Squash*	½ cup	1.3
Sweet potato	1 medium baked	3.4
Turnips*	½ cup	1.6

(*means cooked)

MARCH TO MAY		
Fruit	**Serving Size**	**Fiber (Grams)**
Apricots	3 medium	2.5
Honeydew melon	1 cup	1
Mango	1 medium	3.7
Orange	1 medium	3.1
Pineapple	1 cup	1.9
Strawberries	1 cup	3.4
Vegetables	**Serving Size**	**Fiber (Grams)**
Asparagus*	6 spears	1.4
Broccoli	½ cup	1.3
Collard greens*	1 cup	3.6
Corn*	½ cup	2.3
Green beans*	½ cup	2
Lettuce	½ cup	0.5
Peas*	½ cup	4.4
Spinach	½ cup	0.8
Swiss chard	½ cup	1.8

(*means cooked)

JUNE TO AUGUST		
Fruit	**Serving Size**	**Fiber (Grams)**
Blackberries	½ cup	3.8
Blueberries	1 cup	3.9
Canteloupe	1 cup	1.3
Grapes	1 cup	0.9
Nectarine	1 medium	2.2
Peach	1 medium	1.7
Pear	1 medium	4
Plum	1 medium	1
Rasperries	1 cup	8.4
Strawberries	1 cup	3.4
Watermelon	1 cup	0.8
Vegetables	**Serving Size**	**Fiber (Grams)**
Beets*	½ cup	1.7
Bell pepper	1 medium	1.7
Cucumber	½ cup	0.4
Edamame	½ cup	3.8
Eggplant*	½ cup	1.2
Green beans*	½ cup	2
Lima Beans*	½ cup	6.6
Okra*	½ cup	2.2
Tomatoes	1 medium	1.4
Zucchini*	½ cup	1.3

(*means cooked)

YEAR ROUND		
Fruit/Vegetables	**Serving Size**	**Fiber (Grams)**
Apple	1 medium	3.7
Avocado	½ medium	4.2
Banana	1 medium	2.7
Bell pepper	1 medium	1.7
Cabbage	½ cup	0.8
Carrot	1 medium	2.2
Celery	1 stalk	0.7
Lettuce	½ cup	0.5
Mushrooms	½ cup	0.4
Onion	½ medium	1.4
Papaya	1 medium	5.5
Potato	1 medium	4.8

(*means cooked)

Standard U.S./Metric Measurement Conversions

VOLUME CONVERSIONS

U.S. Volume Measure	Metric Equivalent
⅛ teaspoon	0.5 milliliter
¼ teaspoon	1 milliliter
½ teaspoon	2 milliliters
1 teaspoon	5 milliliters
½ tablespoon	7 milliliters
1 tablespoon (3 teaspoons)	15 milliliters
2 tablespoons (1 fluid ounce)	30 milliliters
¼ cup (4 tablespoons)	60 milliliters
⅓ cup	90 milliliters
½ cup (4 fluid ounces)	125 milliliters
⅔ cup	160 milliliters
¾ cup (6 fluid ounces)	180 milliliters
1 cup (16 tablespoons)	250 milliliters
1 pint (2 cups)	500 milliliters
1 quart (4 cups)	1 liter (about)

WEIGHT CONVERSIONS

U.S. Weight Measure	Metric Equivalent
½ ounce	15 grams
1 ounce	30 grams
2 ounces	60 grams
3 ounces	85 grams
¼ pound (4 ounces)	115 grams
½ pound (8 ounces)	225 grams
¾ pound (12 ounces)	340 grams
1 pound (16 ounces)	454 grams

OVEN TEMPERATURE CONVERSIONS

Degrees Fahrenheit	Degrees Celsius
200 degrees F	95 degrees C
250 degrees F	120 degrees C
275 degrees F	135 degrees C
300 degrees F	150 degrees C
325 degrees F	160 degrees C
350 degrees F	180 degrees C
375 degrees F	190 degrees C
400 degrees F	205 degrees C
425 degrees F	220 degrees C
450 degrees F	230 degrees C

BAKING PAN SIZES

American	Metric
8 x 1½ inch round baking pan	20 x 4 cm cake tin
9 x 1½ inch round baking pan	23 x 3.5 cm cake tin
11 x 7 x 1½ inch baking pan	28 x 18 x 4 cm baking tin
13 x 9 x 2 inch baking pan	30 x 20 x 5 cm baking tin
2 quart rectangular baking dish	30 x 20 x 3 cm baking tin
15 x 10 x 2 inch baking pan	30 x 25 x 2 cm baking tin (Swiss roll tin)
9 inch pie plate	22 x 4 or 23 x 4 cm pie plate
7 or 8 inch springform pan	18 or 20 cm springform or loose bottom cake tin
9 x 5 x 3 inch loaf pan	23 x 13 x 7 cm or 2 lb narrow loaf or pate tin
1½ quart casserole	1.5 liter casserole
2 quart casserole	2 liter casserole

Index